Psychoph
Schi:

GH00336819

Authors:

Dr. Jogin H. Thakore, PhD, MRCPI, MRCPsych
Senior Lecturer in Psychiatry
Consultant Psychiatrist

Patricia Walsh MB, MICGP, MRCPsych
Clinical Research Fellow in Psychiatry

Leona Spelman MB, MRCPsych
Clinical Research Fellow in Psychiatry

Neuroscience Centre
St. Vincent's Hospital
Richmond Road, Dublin 3
Ireland

Sandpiper Publishing
Blackwater Lodge Shop Lane
East Mersea Colchester
Essex CO5 8TR

Tel: +44 (0) 1206 382271
Fax: +44 (0) 1206 382271
E Mail: salmonese@btinternet.com
www.sandpiperpublishing.com

ISBN 0-9538606-2-0

Introduction

With the number of psychopharmacology books currently available it was not without some trepidation that my co-authors and I decided to write this book. Our aim was to provide a concise handbook that would explain some of the theoretical background underlying the usage of antipsychotics and how to treat those suffering from schizophrenia. The latter is of immense importance as it is critical that psychiatric trainees involved in prescribing psychotropic medication are given guidance on how best to use the currently available range of anti-psychotics.

Up to quite recently we had the conventional neuroleptics which were the main-stay for the treatment of schizophrenia. Whilst efficacious in over two thirds of those with the disorder, they were primarily useful in the treatment of positive symptoms such as, hallucinations and delusions. In a sense they revolutionised the manner in which patients were treated when they were introduced in the late 1950s. Not only were the patients relieved of their disturbing symptoms but they had greater options in terms of where they might live as institutions began opening their doors and letting patients settle within the community. Unfortunately, there was a price to pay for this new found symptom-free state and that was the occurrence of various adverse effects, most commonly, extrapyramidal symptoms (EPS). These neurological consequences not only decreased the quality of life of patients but also made them reluctant to take their medications.

New hope has been found with the introduction of atypical antipsychotics. These agents do not, in general, have a propensity for antagonising dopamine type 2 receptors and therefore are relatively free of the EPS seen with conventional neuroleptics. Indeed, these agents appear to work on a broader range of symptoms (positive, negative and cognitive symptoms). Yet, these newer agents have side effects, which in a sense may serve to differentiate one from the other. Though experience with some of these compounds is still relatively limited it would appear that they have much to offer.

Foreword

Schizophrenia is undoubtedly the most disabling of all psychiatric disorders and in global terms probably results in more misery than any other medical condition. Given the high prevalence of the disorder and the fact that it afflicts young people, often resulting in lifetime social and occupational handicap, the economic impact is enormous. In spite of this, many health services in affluent western countries seriously under-resource the services provided to those with psychotic illness and this fact together with the stigma associated with mental illness impacts significantly on sufferers and their families.

On a positive note research into schizophrenia has shown major strides in recent years in terms of epidemiology, genetics, pharmacology and psycho-social interventions. Following the discovery of chlorpromazine by Charpentier and haloperidol by Jannsen in the 1950s pharmacology made limited progress in the subsequent 40 years, with the exception of the development of depot medications. The latter are undoubtedly of major benefit to some patients. The next major landmark in pharmacology was the increased understanding of clozapine in terms of clinical impact and receptor profile. Such understanding resulted in the emergence of atypical antipsychotics. These agents are an advance on traditional medications, not just in terms of decreased side-effects but in terms of therapeutic efficacy. Clinical trials demonstrate benefits in schizophrenic patients with negative symptoms, depressive symptoms and to some extent in patients with cognitive impairment.

The production of this concise handbook by Jogin Thakore and his colleagues is timely. The book reviews the diagnostic classification of schizophrenia and also recent developments in the basic and clinical pharmacology of the disorder. It is an excellent volume with a wealth of information and should be of help especially to those training for the MRCPsych examination, though many consultants will find it a useful update. Nurses and psychologists working with patients who suffer from schizophrenia will also view the book as useful.

Jogin Thakore trained in psychiatry and also completed a PhD in the University of London. He was formerly a senior lecturer at St. Bartholomew's and the Royal Hospital Medical School, London and is currently senior lecturer in psychiatry at the Royal College of Surgeons in Dublin where he heads a very active research team. He has co-authored the book with 2 of his research colleagues, Leona Spelman and Patricia Walsh. As both of these researchers have had recent experience in passing the MRCPsych examination they bring this valuable experience to their writing of the book. If the work helps some doctors in providing better pharmacological interventions for patients with schizophrenia it will be a significant achievement.

Ted Dinan
Department of Pharmacology and Therapeutics
University College Cork

Contents

Chapter 1
Diagnosis and Classification of Schizophrenia
       Leona Spelman   1

Chapter 2
The relevance of Neuronal Receptors to Antipsychotic Drug Action
       Jogin H Thakore   15

Chapter 3
Pharmacology of Conventional and Atypical Antipsychotics
       Patricia Walsh   31

Chapter 4
Adverse Effects of Anti-psychotic Medication
       Leona Spelman   51

Chapter 5
Psychopharmacological Management of Schizophrenia
       Leona Spelman   73

CHAPTER 1 – Leona Spelman

Diagnosis and Classification of Schizophrenia

Schizophrenia is a major psychiatric disorder with onset in early adulthood, characterised by bizarre delusions, auditory hallucinations, strange behaviour and a progressive decline in personal, domestic, social and occupational competence, all occurring in clear consciousness.

Historically, schizophrenia has been defined by symptoms. This view of schizophrenia gives us a narrow definition that does not acknowledge the true heterogenous nature of this disorder. Having said this, it is also important to make sense of the range of symptoms that present to us as clinicians, so that we can classify the condition that requires treatment. Classification systems can identify subtypes of the disorder, direct treatment plans and inform decisions about prognosis.

There are no diagnostic tests available. The two major operational diagnostic systems in use today come from the American Psychiatric Association's Diagnostic and Statistical Manual-IV (1994) and the World Health Organisation Tenth Revision of the International Classification of Diseases ICD-10 (1992). To make a diagnosis of schizophrenia, the clinician must elicit clear evidence of symptoms of psychosis (cross-sectional criteria) and these symptoms must be present for a minimal duration (longitudinal criteria). Schizophrenia is a heterogenous condition. The illness tends to run a prolonged course and the individual patient's symptoms vary throughout different phases of the illness.

Diagnosis of schizophrenia is based on thorough psychiatric evaluation and observation, in order to elicit symptoms that are characteristic of this illness. In order to ensure reliable and valid diagnostic systems, collaboration is required between experts in the area to reach a consensus. This consensus has been achieved through the worldwide scientific collaboration that formulated the classification systems in use today.

Historical Perspective

It is always important to be aware of what history can teach us about contemporary practice. The evolution of the classification of psychiatric illness, as enumerated below, leads us to the systems we have in place today. In the 19th century psychiatrists attempted to classify mental illness. For instance, in 1856, Morel coined the term "demence precoce", to describe an adolescent patient who had lapsed into a withdrawn, silent state having once been bright and active. In 1893, Kraepelin divided the various forms of mental illness into two groupings on the basis of their long-term course. "Dementia praecox" included hebephrenia, catatonia and dementia paranoides and was a progressive disease that pursued a downhill course leading to a chronic illness or at best only partial recovery. The second grouping was termed "manic-depressive insanity", this condition pursued a fluctuating course with frequent relapses, with full recovery after each relapse.

Bleuler coined the term schizophrenia, meaning 'split mind' in 1911. He described the 'fundamental symptoms' of thought disorder, blunting or incongruity of affect, autism and the pervasive ambivalence of the disorder. These symptoms are consistent with simple schizophrenia. Hallucinations, delusions and catatonic phenomenon were considered to be accessory symptoms of less importance.

In 1959, Kurt Schneider focused his attention on the acute phase of the illness in order to clarify a system for the diagnosis of schizophrenia. He described a number of 'symptoms of the first rank' which he considered to be diagnostic of schizophrenia in the absence of overt brain disease, however he accepted that these symptoms were not pathognomonic of the disorder. Therefore, he also described 'symptoms of the second rank' which included hallucinations and delusions of other kinds, perplexity and emotional blunting. 'Schneiderian' symptoms are easy to define so that if they are present they are significant. It is important to consider that 20% of patients with schizophrenia have never had any first rank symptoms. These symptoms do not predict the long-term course of the illness.

Kurt Schneider's 'symptoms of the first rank'

1. Auditory hallucinations taking any one of three specific forms:
   a. Voices repeating the subject's thoughts out loud (Gedankenlautwerden or echo de la pensee, or anticipating his thoughts.)
   b. Two or more hallucinatory voices discussing the subject, or arguing about him, referring to him in the third person.
   c. Voices commenting on the subject's thoughts or behaviour, often as a running commentary.

2. The sensation of alien thoughts being put into the subject's mind by some external agency, or of his own thoughts being taken away (thought insertion or withdrawal).

Kurt Schneider's 'symptoms of the first rank' (cont'd)

3. The sensation that the subject's thinking is no longer confined within his own mind, but is instead shared by, or accessible to, others (thought broadcasting).

4. The sensation of feelings, impulses or acts being experienced or carried out under external control, so that the patient feels as if he were being hypnotised, or had become a robot.

5. The experience of being a passive and reluctant recipient of bodily sensation imposed by some external agency (somatic passivity).

6. Primary delusions.
   Delusional perception – a delusion arising fully fledged on the the basis of a genuine perception which others would regard as commonplace and unrelated.

The lack of consensus on the diagnostic criteria for schizophrenia and the low reliability of psychiatric diagnoses generally, led to a widespread realisation that key terms like schizophrenia must be operationally defined. Schizophrenia is a syndrome. The symptoms present in the acute phase of the syndrome do not predict the course of the illness, which can vary widely. There is not any single agreed definition of schizophrenia and as psychiatry progressed in the late 20th century, psychiatrists focussed on the subtypes of the disorder.

Schizophrenia – a heterogenous disorder

Fish first described the concepts of positive and negative symptoms of mental illness in the 19th century and in the 1980s Crow developed these concepts in relation to schizophrenia. He proposed that there are two pathological processes at play – the positive/negative dichotomy.

> **Type I** *schizophrenia* (positive syndrome) is characterised by acute onset, positive symptoms (delusions, hallucinations and thought disorder), normal ventricles and a good response to medication, thought to be associated with increased dopaminergic activity.

> **Type II** *schizophrenia* (negative syndrome) presents with insidious onset, negative symptoms (apathy, affective flattening and poverty of speech), enlarged ventricles, poor response to medication and a deteriorating course.

This theory was examined and refined by Liddle who examined the phenomenology of the disorder during the chronic phase. He defined three distinguishable clinical syndromes in schizophrenia. The negative symptoms clustering together in a syndrome called psychomotor poverty. The positive symptoms fall into two categories of disorganisation and reality distortion. The characteristic symptoms are as follows:

> *Psychomotor poverty:* poverty of speech, affective flattening, decreased spontaneous movement and poor expressive gestures.

> *Disorganisation:* disorder of the form of thought, incoherent speech and inappropriate affect.

> *Reality distortion:* delusions and hallucinations.

Liddle's classification has been lent credence by neuropsychological studies, which show that each syndrome above is characterised by a specific pattern of test performance and by a specific pattern of regional cerebral blood flow.

In the 1990's research focused on the neuropsychology of schizophrenia. Kraepelin, in 1893, introduced the concept of cognitive decline in schizophrenia with his description of 'dementia praecox'. It is now universally accepted that schizophrenia is a brain disease that disrupts the normal functioning of many cognitive abilities. 25% of patients demonstrate impairment of memory. 50% of patients perform poorly on tests of executive function. There is evidence of emotion recognition deficit, which correlates with the severity of positive and negative symptoms. Almost two-thirds of patients with schizophrenia perform poorly, compared to control subjects, on tests of attention. Verbal memory, executive function and selective attention appear to predict the level of a patient's overall function in the community. Therefore cognitive deficits contribute to the impairment in social and occupational functioning that is inherent in the psychopathology of schizophrenia.

The classification of schizophrenia is of vital importance, as one can see from the preceding discussion. The range of symptoms with which your patient presents will dictate the antipsychotic medication you decide to prescribe. Typical antipsychotic drugs do not improve any of the cognitive deficits seen in schizophrenia. In contrast atypical antipsychotic drugs improve a number of the deficits associated with schizophrenia.

Classification systems – Contemporary practice

The most widely used definitions of schizophrenia are the American Psychiatric Association's DSM-IV and World Health Organisation's 1992 ICD-10. These diagnostic classifications are commonly used to define schizophrenia for research purposes and define the subtype and course of the condition. These classification systems differ as to the minimal duration of illness in order to make a diagnosis (see table).

While assessing the patient, the clinician must be aware of the neurological conditions that can mimic schizophrenia, such as temporal lobe epilepsy and central nervous system neoplasm. Drugs such as amphetamines, lysergic acid and ecstasy can all produce symptoms of schizophrenia, that usually resolve with abstinence from the drug. Schizophrenia may be diagnosed in patients who describe persistent psychotic symptoms six months after abstinence from the drug. Affective symptoms are often present in individuals with a diagnosis of schizophrenia. To make a diagnosis of schizophrenia, affective symptoms must not be prominent.

Criteria for schizophrenia in DSM-IV

A. Characteristic symptoms of the active phase
Two (or more) of the following, each present for a significant portion of time during a one-month period (or less if successfully treated)
1) Delusions
2) Hallucinations
3) Disorganised speech (e.g. frequent derailment or incoherence)
4) Grossly disorganised or catatonic behaviour
5) Negative symptoms, i.e. affective flattening, alogia, or avolition

Criteria for schizophrenia in DSM-IV (cont'd)

B. Social / occupational dysfunction
For a significant portion of the time since the onset of the disturbance, one or more major areas of functioning such as work, interpersonal relations, or self-care are markedly below the level achieved prior to the onset (or when the onset is in childhood or adolescence, failure to achieve expected level of interpersonal, academic, or occupational achievement)

C. Duration
Continuous signs of the disturbance persist for at least six months. This six-month period must include at least one month of symptoms (or less if successfully treated) that meet criterion A (i.e. active-phase symptoms) and may include periods of prodromal or residual symptoms. During these prodromal or residual periods, the signs of the disturbance may be manifested by only negative symptoms or by two or more symptoms listed in criterion A present in an attenuated form (e.g. odd beliefs, unusual perceptual experiences)

D. Schizoaffective and mood disorder exclusion
Schizoaffective disorder and mood disorder with psychotic features have been ruled out because either (i) no major depressive, manic, or mixed episodes have occurred concurrently with the active-phase symptoms, or (ii) if mood episodes have occurred during active-phase symptoms, their total duration has been brief relative to the duration of the active and residual periods.

Criteria for schizophrenia in DSM-IV (cont'd)

E. Substance/general medical condition exclusion
The disturbance is not due to the direct physiological effects of a substance (e.g. a drug of abuse, a medication) or a general medical condition.

F. Relationship to a pervasive developmental disorder
If there is a history of autistic disorder or another pervasive development disorder, the additional diagnosis of schizophrenia is made only if prominent delusions or hallucinations are also present for at least one month (or less if successfully treated).

Symptomatic criteria for Schizophrenia in ICD-10

The normal requirements for a diagnosis of schizophrenia is that a minimum of one very clear symptom (and usually two or more if less clear-cut) belonging to any one of the groups listed as (a)-(d) below, or symptoms from at least two of the groups referred to as (e)-(h), should have been clearly present for most of the time during a period of one month or more.

(a) Thought echo, thought insertion or withdrawal and thought broadcasting.

(b) Delusions of control, influence, or passivity, clearly referred to body or limb.

(c) Movements or specific thoughts, actions, or sensations; delusional perception.

(d) Hallucinatory voices giving a running commentary on the patient's behaviour, or discussing the patient among themselves, or other types of hallucinatory voices coming from some part of the body.

(e) Persistent delusions of other kinds that are culturally inappropriate and completely impossible.

(f) Persistent hallucinations in any modality, when accompanied either by fleeting or half-formed delusions without clear affective content, or by persistent over-valued ideas, or when occurring every day for weeks or months on end.

Symptomatic criteria for Schizophrenia in ICD-10 (cont'd)

(g) Breaks or interpolations in the train of thought, resulting in incoherence or irrelevant speech, or neologisms.

(h) Catatonic behaviour, such as excitement, posturing, or waxy flexibility, negativism, mutism and stupor.

(i) 'Negative' symptoms such as marked apathy, paucity of speech and blunting or incongruity of emotional responses, usually resulting in social withdrawal and lowering of social performance; it must be clear that these are not due to depression or to neuroleptic medication.

(j) A significant and consistent change in the overall quality of some aspects of personal behaviour, manifest as loss of interest, aimlessness, idleness, a self-absorbed attitude and social withdrawal.

Classification of subtypes of schizophrenia	
DSM-IV	**ICD-10**
Paranoid	Paranoid
Disorganised	Hebephrenic
Catatonic	Catatonic
Undifferentiated	Undifferentiated
Residual	Residual
	Simple schizophrenia
	Post-schizophrenia depression
	Other schizophrenia
	Unspecified schizophrenia

In summary, these classification systems, though the standard systems in use today, perhaps have fallen behind the research findings of recent years. It is important to be knowledgable about these classification systems in terms of standardising diagnoses. In turn, it is important to recognise that our knowledge of the neuro-biology of schizophrenia is improving. To recognise the historical perspective in the classification of schizophrenia informs us that our understanding is constantly evolving. With this evolution, in the recognition of the cognitive deficit state in schizophrenia, our treatments should change in tandem. Further treatment developments should look to the key symptoms of this complex disorder.

References

American Psychiatric Association.
Diagnostic and statistical manual of mental disorders (4th edn).
Am Psych Assoc, Washington, DC.1994.

World Health Organisation.
The ICD-10 classification of mental and behavioural disorders.
World Health Organisation, Geneva, 1992.

Kohler CG, Bilker W, Hagendoorn M, *et al.*
Emotion recognition deficit in schizophrenia: association with
symptomatology and cognition.
Biol Psych 2000; 48(2): 127-136.

Heinrichs RW, Zakzanis KK.
Neurocognitive deficit in schizophrenia.
A quantitative review of the evidence.
Neuropsych 1998; 12: 426-445.

Green MF.
What are the functional consequences of neurocognitive deficits
in schizophrenia?
Am J of Psych 1996; 153: 321-330.

Meltzer HY, McGurk SR.
The effects of clozapine, risperidone and olanzapine on cognitive
function in schizophrenia.
Schizo Bull 1999; 25: 233-255.

Tsuang MT, Simpson JC, Kronfold Z.
Subtypes of drug abuse with psychosis.
Arch of Gen Psych 1982; 39: 141-147

The Relevance of Neuronal Receptors to Antipsychotic Drug Action

Introduction

The pace of change regarding the characterisation of known and novel neurotransmitter systems is fast and at times difficult to keep up with. Molecular pharmacology offers us the prospect of delineating and understanding not only receptors but also the neuro-chemicals and their pathways with a view to appreciating 'normal' brain function and shedding light on potential pathophysiological mechanisms. Therefore, psychopharmacology not only refers to the compounds that we use to treat disorders of the brain but also to the study of the biological processes that may be responsible for normal or aberrant central nervous system function. Therefore, the intent of this chapter is to introduce various neuronal receptor systems and their relevance in terms of potential antipsychotic drug action. For the sake of brevity, this chapter discusses only 3 neurochemical systems namely, dopamine (DA), serotonin (5HT) and the excitatory amino acid, glutamate.

Each neurotransmitter is discussed in terms of:

1. Brief introduction.
2. Anatomical pathways.
3. Biochemical processes.
4. Receptor systems.
5. Evidence leading to implicating its role in schizophrenia.
6. The relevance of it's function in terms of antipsychotic drug action.

Dopamine

Of all the neuronal systems which may be involved in schizophrenia, DA has received by far the most attention. Initially, it was found that patients with Parkinson's disease, a neurological disorder associated with a decrease in nigrostriatal DA levels, had various extrapyramidal symptoms including akinesia, rigidity and tremor. Keen observation led to early researchers to conclude that patients given chlorpromazine suffered from these symptoms as side-effects, leading to the observation that antipsychotics may act by blocking DA function. In a sense, these findings led to generation of the DA hypothesis of schizophrenia.

Dopamine Pathways.

The cell bodies of DA are labelled A1-12 though most of these are found in the A9 nucleus.

1. Nigrostriatal pathway – the vast majority of the cell bodies are found within the A9 nucleus which is located in the substantia nigra and run onto the striatum (caudate nucleus & putamen) and amygdala.

2. Mesolimbic pathway – Cell bodies originate from the A10 nucleus and innervates the nucleus accumbens, olfactory tubercle and parts of the cortex (mesocortical system), for example the prefrontal and perirhinal cortex.

3. Fibres from the A12 nucleus (located within the arcuate nucleus of the hypothalamus) travel the short distance to the pituitary gland where DA controls the release of prolactin (the action is inhibitory).

Biochemistry of DA

Tyrosine is synthesised from phenylalanine in the liver and is actively transported into the brain. It is metabolised by a variety of means and the final product is homovanillic acid (Fig. 1).

Fig .1
The biosynthetic pathway for DA

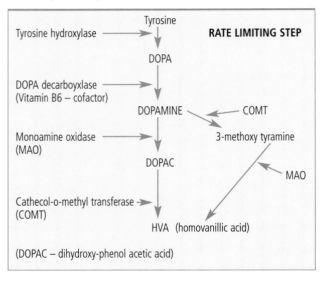

DA receptors

There are 5 types of DA receptors, namely, D1, D2, D3, D4 and D5. In terms of drug sensitivity and structure, D1 and D5 are categorised together and termed, 'D1-like' and D2, D3 and D4 are categorised together and termed, 'D2-like'. D1 receptors bind to and stimulate adenylate cyclase (second messenger system) while D2 receptors have the opposite effect. The location of each of the 5 subtypes also differs; D1 receptors are located predominantly in the cortex, D2 receptors in the striatum and limbic structures while D3 receptors are found in the nucleus accumbens.

Dopamine Hypothesis of Schizophrenia

Though there is much evidence supporting this contention it is by no means unequivocal:

1. Effective antipsychotics block D2 receptors.

2. Amphetamine, which release DA from presynaptic neurones can precipitate psychotic episodes in normal volunteers and patients with schizophrenia.

3. Post mortem studies and Positron Emission Tomography (PET) studies have revealed increased D2 receptor concentrations yet these findings have not been supported by studies in drug naive patients with schizophrenia, implying that the changes seen may have been secondary to prior antipsychotic usage.

4. Imaging studies have indicated that patients with schizophrenia have 'hypofrontality', in that there is reduced cerebral blood flow during certain tasks of cognitive function (e.g. Wisconsin Card Sorting test) suggesting a relative deficit of DA function in this particular brain area (prefrontal cortex).

Clinical relevance of DA neurotransmission in terms of antipsychotic action

Dopamine systems are one of the primary targets for antipsychotics drugs, be they conventional or atypical. Indeed, antipsychotic agents acting on mesolimbic and mesocortical tracts are believed to be responsible for the therapeutic effect of these compounds while occupancy of the tuberoinfundibular tract can result in hyperprolactinaemia and various endocrine disturbances.

Of the 5 DA receptors mentioned, the D2 receptor is by far the most important, at present, though the location of D3 offers a tantalising prospect for future drug action. D1 receptors are blocked by antipsychotics (D1 receptors are bound with high affinity by conventional antipsychotics and with low affinity by atypical neuroleptics) yet to differing extents. Yet, it would appear that atypical antipsychotics increase DA levels in the prefrontal area which may explain their beneficial effects in patients with negative symptoms.

Depolarisation inactivation is the means by which antipsychotics are believed to act, in that they prevent the repolarisation (allowing them to be able to depolarise to further action potentials) of dopaminergic neurones in the mesolimbic area (ventral tegmental) following chronic treatment. Imaging studies have indicated that approximately 70% of D2 receptors are occupied by therapeutic concentrations of any antipsychotic drug. Therefore, using higher than recommended doses in the vast majority of patients confer little extra benefit though would probably increase the likelihood of adverse effects.

With this in mind, the degree to which an antipsychotic binds, 'loosely or tightly' (relative to endogenous dopamine, which competes with the drug for receptor occupancy), determines whether it is less or more likely (respectively) to induce extrapyramidal symptoms (EPS) (e.g. tremor, akathesia) (Table 1). Therefore, using lower doses of drugs which bind tightly and higher doses of drugs which bind loosely should result in minimal amounts of EPS.

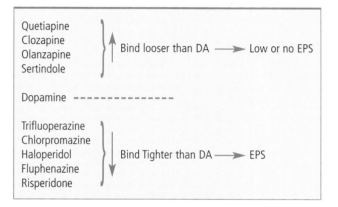

Serotonin

The discovery that lysergic acid diethylamine (LSD) and psilocybin, both of which are psychomimetics, increase serotonergic drive prompted the study of the role of the indoleamine, 5HT, in the pathogenesis of schizophrenia. Much of the recent interest in 5HT has also arisen as a result of the findings that potent atypical antipsychotics such as clozapine have greater 5HT2-D2 binding ratios which may explain their reduced propensity to cause EPS.

Serotonin Pathways

Cell bodies of 5HT are located in the brainstem (midbrain and upper pons) and are labelled B1-9, and are termed the raphe nuclei. The serotonergic system not only releases 5HT at synapses but also has the ability to release 5HT from axonal varicosities in non-synaptic areas therefore, increasing its area of influence greatly.

1. The B7 and B8 nuclei project upwards to the forebrain to the hypothalamus, olfactory complex, caudate nucleus, hippocampus and cortex.

2. The caudal projection from the raphe nuclei terminate in the trigeminal nucleus, and the dorsal and ventral horns of the spinal cord.

Biochemistry of 5HT

L-tryptophan, the precursor for 5HT is found in the diet and is actively transported into the brain. It is metabolised following uptake into the presynaptic neurone and the final product is 5-hydroxyindole acetic acid (Fig. 2).

Biochemistry of 5HT

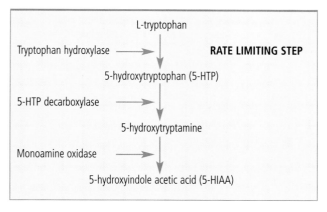

L-tryptophan

Tryptophan hydroxylase ⟶ **RATE LIMITING STEP**

5-hydroxytryptophan (5-HTP)

5-HTP decarboxylase ⟶

5-hydroxytryptamine

Monoamine oxidase ⟶

5-hydroxyindole acetic acid (5-HIAA)

5HT Receptors

There are 7 families of 5HT receptors with further subdivisions within each major category, namely; 5HT1 (subtypes - a, b, c, d, e, f), 5HT2 (subtypes - a, b ,c), 5HT3, 5HT4, 5HT5, 5HT6, 5HT7. Of these the first 3 are best categorised. The 5HT1 is located in the spinal cord and hippocampal cortex and is coupled with the adenylate cyclase second messenger system. The 5HT2a and 5HT2c receptors are part of the G protein superfamily whose activation leads to the activation of phospholipase C and hydrolysis of phosphoinositide. The 5HT2a receptor is located in a number of brain regions including the frontal, parietal and cingulate cortices, and the hypothalamus, caudate-puta-men and nucleus accumbens. The 5HT2c receptor is found amongst other areas, in the choroid plexus, cingulate gyrus, substantia nigra and nucleus accumbens. The 5HT3 receptor is the only known ligand gated 5HT receptor and is found in the lower brain stem, amygdala, hippocampus and nucleus tractus solitarius.

Serotonin Hypothesis of Schizophrenia

This theory has arisen as a result of the observations that LSD and psilocybin can cause symptoms similar to schizophrenia in healthy individuals and precipitate psychotic episodes in those with, or prone to, schizophrenia. Evidence which supports and refutes this hypothesis is:

1. The newer antipsychotics, which are highly effective, such as olanzapine and clozapine are potent 5HT2 antagonists with data suggesting that these agents have a greater potency at the 5HT2a/c sites than at the D2 receptor.

2. Plasma levels of 5HT are elevated in patients with schizophrenia.

3. Some, though not all, studies have found CSF levels of 5-HIAA (5-hydroxy indoleacetic acid) to be raised in patients with schizophrenia and this in turn was found to correlate with certain symptoms such as delusions.

4. Though LSD can induce psychotic symptoms, it tends to produce perceptual abnormalities such as visual hallucinations which are not a characteristic feature of schizophrenia.

Clinical relevance of 5HT neurotransmission in terms of antipsychotic action

Antagonism of the 5HT2a receptor in particular appears to be a critical characteristic of atypical antipsychotics which may help explain their greater efficacy and reduced propensity to produce EPS. Alleviation of depressive symptoms by this class of antipsychotics may also be due to the fact that they antagonise this class of 5HT receptor. 5HT2c receptors appear to exert a tonic inhibitory control over frontocortical DA release and therefore their blockade by atypical agents would increase DA levels which in turn may explain their greater efficacy in negative symptoms. However, a potential disadvantage of blocking 5HT2 receptors is a propensity to increase appetite and therefore induce weight gain, though against this argument is the observation that not all atypical agents cause significant increases in body mass index.

5HT3 receptors may be involved in the actions of atypical antipsychotics as indicated by the ability of these agents to inhibit the release of mesolimbic and striatal DA release.

Excitatory Amino Acids

The psychomimetic effects of phencyclidine (PCP) were known of 40 years ago; it was found that PCP provoked a relatively prolonged psychosis in those with schizophrenia. In addition it was shown that PCP blocked the glutamate receptor and could induce both positive and negative symptoms in normal individuals. Several neuro-excitatory amino acids possess neurotransmitter properties though evidence favours glutamate as being the most important.

Glutamatergic Pathways

Over 60% of all synapses in the brain use glutamate as their neuro-transmitter and it is probably used by all excitatory pathways within the CNS. In fact, the cerebral cortex and higher brain centres contain the highest amount of glutamate found anywhere within the CNS. Due to its widespread distribution, it is difficult to single out any particular systems though some are noteworthy:

1. The anterior cingulate gyrus receives it's glutamatergic tracts from a number of intrinsic (pyramidal layers) and extrinsic sources, including the subcortex (e.g. thalamus) and the amygdala.

2. The hippocampus projects to the lateral septum and nucleus accumbens.

3. Corticofugal tracts include those from the frontal cortex to DA rich areas such as the striatum, substantia nigra and nucleus accumbens.

Biochemistry of Glutamate

Most of the glutamate that acts as a neurotransmitter is principally synthesised from glutamine though there are potentially 6 other means by which it may be produced. Glutamate is taken up by astrocytes and converted into glutamine by glutamine synthetase. After diffusing out of the astrocyte it is taken up by nerve terminals and within mitochondria is converted to glutamate by glutaminase. In turn, glutamate released by the nerve terminal is taken up actively into presynaptic neurones and glia and converted into glutamine by glutamine synthetase.

Glutamatergic receptors

These are divided into those that use ion channels (ionotropic) or traditional second messenger systems (metabotropic) (Table 2).

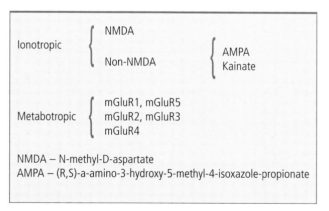

Ionotropic
- NMDA
- Non-NMDA
  - AMPA
  - Kainate

Metabotropic
- mGluR1, mGluR5
- mGluR2, mGluR3
- mGluR4

NMDA – N-methyl-D-aspartate
AMPA – (R,S)-a-amino-3-hydroxy-5-methyl-4-isoxazole-propionate

The non-NMDA glutamate receptors, AMPA and kainate are composed of a channel through which Na+ and K+ may pass. The AMPA receptors are principally located within the outer layers of the cortex, lateral septum and cerebellum. Kainate receptors are found primarily within hippocampus, deep cortical layers and thalamus. NMDA receptors are ligand gated channels (Na+, K+ and Ca++) and are usually co-localised with non-NMDA sites, implying that they may amplify the effects of glutamate.

Glutamatergic hypothesis of Schizophrenia

Excitotoxic processes may be involved in the pathogenesis of schizo-phrenia. As mentioned earlier, PCP non-competitively binds to NMDA receptors and is psychomimetic. In addition, it appears that patients with schizophrenia have an increased number of NMDA sites in the frontal cortex. CSF levels of glutamate are lower in patients with schizophrenia than in normal individuals. Yet, levels of this excitatory amino acid have been found to be reduced in the frontal cortex and hippocampus which would be out of keeping with diminished activity of this system in these areas. This may have implications from a neurodevelopmental perspective, as glutamate stimulates synapto-genesis and maturation of synapses in the developing brain.

Lastly, interactions between DA and the glutamatergic system have been hypothesised. For instance, glutamate appears to increase striatal DA release via the NMDA receptor, providing evidence that the dopaminergic overactivity seen in schizophrenia may in fact be an epiphenomenon of glutamatergic dysfunction.

Clinical relevance of glutamatergic neurotransmission in terms of antipsychotic action

The major difficulty in developing agents that act directly upon the glutamatergic system is their propensity to cause memory impairments and other serious neurotoxic effects such as catatonia and seizures. Therefore, agents that indirectly modulate the NMDA receptor such as D-cycloserine can be potentially used as antipsychotic compounds when added to a stable antipsychotic regimen (clozapine), D-cycloserine has been shown to improve not only the positive and negative symptoms of schizophrenia but also various neuropsychological deficits associated with this illness.

Conclusion

This chapter is by no means comprehensive in terms of covering all potential neurotransmitters systems which may be involved in schizophrenia. With this in mind, conventional neurotransmitters do antagonise histaminergic sites thereby inducing sedation and possibly weight gain and also block adrenergic receptors leading to hypotension and sexual dysfunction. As it is unlikely that either of these 2 systems plays a role in the pathogenesis of schizophrenia or indeed, further explain how antipsychotics act, they have not been discussed in this chapter. Anticholinergic effects of conventional neuroleptics lead to various unpleasant symptoms such as dry mouth and blurred vision. It would appear that antimuscarinics used in conjunction with conventional agents merely reduce related adverse effects but do not appear to have intrinsic antipsychotic properties per se.

Therefore, the 3 neuronal systems discussed are important in terms of the psychopharmacology of schizophrenia . However, it is likely that an interplay between DA, 5HT and glutamate and other peptides, or indeed other amines, may better explain the phenomenon of schizophrenia and the efficacy of the agents currently used to treat this condition.

References

Meltzer HY, Matsubara S, Lee JC.
Classification of typical and atypical drugs on the basis of dopamine
D-1, D-2 and serotonin pKi values.
J Pharmacol Exp Ther1989; 251: 238-246.

Lieberman JA, Mailman RB, Duncan G, Sikich L, Chakos MH,
Nichols DE, Kraus J.
Serotonergic basis of antipsychotic drug effects in schizophrenia.
Biol Psychiatry 1998; 44: 1099-1117.

Olney JW, Farber NB.
Glutamate receptor dysfunction and schizophrenia.
Arch Gen Psych 1995; 52: 998-1007.

Seeman P, Tallerico T.
Antipsychotic drugs which elicit little or no parkinsonism bind more
loosely than dopamine to brain D2 receptors, yet occupy high levels
of these receptors.
Mol Psych 1998; 3: 123-134.

Webster RA, Jordan CC. Neurotransmitters, Drugs and Disease.
Blackwell Scientific Publications, London, 1989.

Khan RS, Davis KL.
New Developments in Dopamine and Schizophrenia.
In: Psychopharmacology: The fourth generation of Progress
(eds Bloom FE, Kupfer DJ).
Raven Press, New York, 1995, pp 1193-1204.

Pharmacology of Conventional and Atypical Antipsychotics

Introduction

Though developed by Labroit in 1952 as an anaesthetic agent, chlorpromazine was found to have sedative properties, which prompted Delay and Deniker to use it in patients with psychoses. In a sense, the use of this agent was truly revolutionary as it not only alleviated certain symptoms of psychoses but also allowed the concept of care in the community to develop as it allowed a significant proportion of patients who were once cared for in a custodial setting to live at home, in hostels or independently. Many other drugs have been developed since 1952 and the vast majority of these are termed 'conventional' and are characterised by the fact that they may act by blocking type 2 dopamine (D2) receptors. In the recent past, we have seen the gradual introduction of a separate class of compounds which have been designated 'atypical'. This definition arises from the observation that this class of antipsychotic, whilst being highly effective, induces fewer, if any, extrapyramidal symptoms (EPS). This chapter describes the clinical pharmacology of both conventional and atypical antipsychotics.

Conventional Antipsychotics

Conventional or typical antipsychotics have been the first line treatment for schizophrenia for over half a century. They can be divided, based on the strength of their affinity for the mesolimbic and nigrostriatal dopamine type 2 (D2) receptors, into high, medium and low potency antipsychotics. The degree of D2 receptor blockade in the striatum determines the propensity to develop extrapyramidal side effects (EPS). High potency antipsychotics like haloperidol, which exhibit high D2 blockade, have an increased risk of EPS and low and medium potency antipsychotics, which exhibit lower D2 blockade, have a decreased risk of EPS.

In addition, low potency antipsychotics, like thioridazine, however have more anticholinergic and antihistaminergic side effects at therapeutic doses, which can lead to QT interval prolongation on the ECG, sedation, hypotension, weight gain and seizures. In terms of symptom profiles, typical antipsychotics are effective in the treatment of the positive symptoms of schizophrenia. Unlike atypical antipsychotics, they are, in general, not effective in treating the negative or cognitive symptoms of schizophrenia, which can be disabling. Lastly, exceeding recommended daily dose range leads to little if any therapeutic benefits but significantly increases the risks of EPS.

Classification of conventional antipsychotics

These compounds are generally classified according to their structure (Table 1). Dose equivalencies with respect to chlorpromazine are given in Table 2.

Table 1

I. Phenothiazines
    Aliphatic derivatives   e.g. chlorpromazine.
    Piperidine derivatives e.g. thioridazine.
    Piperazine derivatives e.g. trifluoperazine,
                             fluphenazine decanoate.

II. Butyrophenones   e.g. haloperidol, droperidol.

III. Diphenylbutylpiperidines e.g. pimozide, fluspirelene.

IV. Benzamide   e.g. sulpiride.

V. Thioxanthenes   e.g. zuclopenthixol, flupenthixol.

Phenothiazines

All the phenothiazines have the same three-ring structure but differ in the side chains joined to the nitrogen atom of the middle ring.

1. **Aliphatic side chain derivative**
   Chlorpromazine:
   This is the original antipsychotic and has a wide range of effects on many different transmitter systems leading to a high incidence of adverse effects such as hypotension and sexual dysfunction (antiadrenergic), sedation and weight gain (antihistaminergic). In terms of it's pharmacokinetics, it is well absorbed but undergoes extensive first pass metabolism in the gut wall and liver with hydroxylation, oxidation and conjugation. It is widely distributed and concentrates well in the brain. It is strongly protein bound and undergoes hepatic metabolism. It is eliminated in the urine and intestine as over 150 metabolites (some of which are active), giving it a relatively long half-life which can be up to 12 days. As chlorpromazine is hepatotoxic it is contraindicated in hepatic disease. A Cochrane review showed chlorpromazine to reduce relapse and improve the positive symptoms of schizophrenia, with the usual therapeutic dose ranging from 75-300 mg per day.

2. **Piperidine derivatives**
   Thioridazine:
   Thioridazine is rapidly and completely absorbed from the gastro-intestinal tract. Maximum plasma concentrations are reached 2-4 hours after ingestion. It is eliminated mainly via the faeces but also via the kidney. Plasma elimination half-life is approximately 10 hours. The major problem with thioridazine is that a dose-related increase in risk of lengthened QT interval (which can lead to various ventricular arrhythmias) has been reported, detectable at doses as low as 10mg/day. Due to concerns about QT prolongation, thioridazine is now only approved for the

treatment of resistant schizophrenia. It is considered inappropriate for patients with a history of cardiac arrhythmias (Reilly et al., 2000). Patients commencing thioridazine require a baseline and routine follow up ECGs and serum potassium levels.

If used, the usual amount is 150-600mg in divided doses. However, a maximum daily dose of 800mg/day may be given for a period not exceeding 4 weeks. Lower doses should be used in the elderly.

3. Piperazine derivatives

These are medium to high potency antipsychotics. Due to their receptor binding profiles, they carry a high risk of EPS, sedation (antihistaminergic effects) and a low risk of hypotension and anticholinergic adverse effects such as dry mouth and blurred vision.

Trifluoperazine:

This is widely used as an antipsychotic and is sometimes claimed to have "activating" effects at low doses. Starting dose is 5mg twice daily, increasing after 7 days to 15mg daily. Maximum dose is 25mg.

Fluphenazine:

An oral preparation is available but this is usually used as a depot. This is a high potency antipsychotic. Plasma levels of fluphenazine following fluphenazine injection have shown half-lives of plasma clearance ranging from 2-16 weeks, emphasising the importance of adjusting dose and interval to the individual requirements of each patient. The slow decline in plasma levels means that a reasonably stable plasma level can usually be achieved with injections spaced at 2-4 week intervals.

Perphenazine:

This has a relatively short half-life of 8-12 hours. This is a medium potency antipsychotic. Dose range is 12-24 mg/day.

Butyrophenones
Haloperidol:
This is a high potency agent with low cholinergic, adrenergic, serotonergic and histaminergic binding. However, due to it's keen binding of the D2 site, it is associated with a significant frequency of EPS. First pass metabolism of 40-70% means that oral doses will result in significantly lower levels compared to an equivalent parenteral dose. The main route of elimination is by hepatic gluconidation.
Haloperidol is frequently associated with extrapyramidal symptoms. Haloperidol is the drug of choice in patients with hepatic impairment. Dose range is 1.5-20mg/day.

Droperidol:
This was discontinued world wide in 2001 due to concerns over a dose-related increase in risk of lengthened QT interval (Reilly, 2000).

Diphenylbutylpiperidines
Pimozide:
This is structurally similar to the butyrophenones. It is relatively non-sedating and can be administered in a single daily dose. It appears to selectively block central D2 receptors, but only affects noradrenergic sites at higher doses. Absorption is greater than 50% after oral administration, with peak serum levels occurring 6-8 hours after dosing. It is extensively metabolised, primarily by N-dealkylation in the liver. It has potentially cardiotoxic effects, therefore baseline and routine follow up ECGs are recommended for patients on pimozide. Initial dose is 2-4 mg daily. Maintenance dose is 2-12 mg daily. Maximum dose is 20mg daily.

Fluspirilene:
See under depots.

Substituted Benzamides
Sulpiride:
This antipsychotic primarily antagonises D2 receptors but can also bind D3 and D4 receptors. Despite the potent D2 blockade, the incidence of EPS is much reduced. Peak serum levels are reached 3-6 hours after an oral dose. The plasma half-life is approximately 8 hours. Approximately 45% is bound to plasma proteins. Over 95% of the compound is excreted in the urine and faeces unchanged. Sulpiride is not very lipophilic and therefore higher doses may be required in order to penetrate the blood brain barrier to achieve therapeutic effects.

Predominantly negative symptoms as well as depression respond to doses below 800mg per day, therefore, a starting dose of 400mg twice daily is recommended. Reducing this dose towards 200mg twice daily will normally increase the alerting effects of sulpiride. Mood elevation is observed after a few days of treatment. Initially, patients are commenced on 400-800mg daily in two divided doses and dose is adjusted within a range of 100-1200mg twice daily.

Thioxanthines
Zuclopenthixol:
This compound acts primarily at D2 receptors and is therefore likely to cause EPS, especially if used in high doses. This drug is absorbed slowly, undergoes extensive hepatic metabolism and is renally excreted. It achieves wide tissue distribution, peak levels occur in 3-6 hr and its elimination half life is 24 hr. The usual oral dose is 20-30mg/day, increasing as necessary to a maximum of 150mg/day, in divided doses. The usual maintenance dose in chronic schizophrenia is 20-50mg/day. The dosage may need to be reduced in the elderly due to reduced rates of metabolism and elimination.

Flupenthixol:
See under depots. An oral preparation is also available. Starting oral dose is 3-9 mg per day to a maximum of 18mg/day. Initial dosage may need to be reduced to a quarter or half the normal starting dose in the frail or elderly.

Dibenzoxapines
Loxapine:
This is of similar efficacy to chlorpromazine. There is some evidence that loxapine is an equipotent blocker of 5HT2 and D2 receptors, and hence might be claimed to be atypical, but a Cochrane review concluded that whilst loxapine was an antipsychotic, it was under-researched and had no clear advantages over other typical drugs.

Table 2 **Equivalent Doses of Typical Antipsychotics**	
Drug	**Equivalent Dose**
(Oral preparations)	
Chlorpromazine	100 mg
Haloperidol	3 mg
Trifluoperazine	5 mg
Flupenthixol	3 mg
Zuclopenthixol	25 mg
Sulpiride	200 mg
Fluphenazine	2 mg
Pimozide	2 mg
Loxapine	10 mg
Thioridazine	100 mg
(Intramuscular preparations)	
Fluphenazine decanoate	5 mg/week
Pipothiazine palmitate	10 mg/week
Flupenthixol decanoate	10 mg/week
Zuclopenthixol decanoate	100 mg/week
Haloperidol decanoate	15 mg/week

Intramuscular preparations (depot) of Antipsychotics

Intramuscular administration of antipsychotics is widely used throughout the world. The major advantages are:

1. Assured compliance.

2. Proven reduction in relapses, rehospitalisation and severity of relapse.

3. Reduction in bioavailability problems (some people metabolise antipsychotics extensively via the first pass effect).

4. By being sure of the doses received, depots should be able to facilitate better downward titration of doses so as to reduce the incidence of side effects.

The major disadvantages of depots are:

1. The difficulty of altering a dose acutely if side effects develop.

2. Patients seeing depot administration as being "controlled", having no control over their treatment or, worse still as being a punishment.

Yet, it should not be enough just to prevent relapse with a depot. The Cochrane review of depots noted:

1. The lack of decent trials and low patient numbers used in existing trials.

2. That the incidence of problems and complications, e.g. bleeding or hematoma, leakage, inflammatory nodules etc associated with long-term depot injections, have probably been underreported. The need for a meticulous (z-tracking) injection technique and using the most appropriate dose and preparation for that individual are essential for long-term success.

Depot antipsychotics are long acting esterified antipsychotics that are suspended in a fatty base. They are administered as an intramuscular injection either on a weekly or monthly basis, the frequency being determined by the clinical situation at hand and the type of depot used. As with all oil-based injections, it is important to ensure, by aspiration before injection, that inadvertent intravascular injection does not occur.

The currently available depots are typical antipsychotics but it is anticipated that atypical depots may be available in the near future (Table 3). In patients who have not previously received depot neuroleptics, treatment is usually started with a small test dose in order to assess tolerability, 4-10 days before commencing the patient on full maintenance doses. A quarter to a half of recommended doses should be used in the elderly who may be prone to toxicity, drug interactions and side effects. Control of severe psychotic symptoms may take up to 6 months at an adequate dosage.

When using a depot:
1. The need for depots should be regularly reviewed, given the risk of EPS with typical depots.

2. Patients should be maintained on the lowest effective doses of depot antipsychotics and reducing the interval between doses is not recommended unless absolutely necessary.

3. Since individual response to neuroleptic drugs is variable, dosage should be individually determined and is best initiated and titrated under close clinical supervision.

4. Take note of the fact that it can take up to 6 months for a depot antipsychotic to be excreted from the body.

Types of depots
Haloperidol decanoate
After intramuscular injection, haloperidol decanoate is gradually released from muscle tissue and slowly hydrolysed into free halo- peridol, which enters the systemic circulation. The average elimination half life is 3 weeks. The drug is widely distributed in the body, is strongly protein bound and has a half-life of 12-40 hours. Haloperidol decanoate has little antihistaminergic or anticholinergic activity. It is associated with a high incidence of extrapyramidal side effects and a low incidence of sedation.

An initial dose of 50mg every 4 weeks is recommended, increasing, if necessary by 50mg increments up to 200mg every four weeks. Subsequent monthly doses should be reassessed according to the patient's response. If, for clinical reasons, two-weekly administration is preferred, these doses should be halved. It is probably best reserved for chronic relapsing schizophrenics responsive to halo- peridol.

Zuclopenthixol decanoate
The drug is slowly absorbed. It is extensively metabolised in the liver, widely distributed in tissues with peak levels around 3 to 6 hours and subsequently eliminated with a biological half-life of one day.

The usual dosage range is 200-500mg every one to four weeks. Maximum dosage is 600mg per week. Thioxanthines have a high affinity for D1 and D2 receptors. Zuclopenthixol possesses a marked specific calming effect and a non-specific sedative action.

Flupenthixol decanoate
This is a dopamine specific thioxanthine antipsychotic, with potentially activating effects at low dose and has been dubbed a "partial atypical". The usual dosage lies between 50mg to 200mg every two to four weeks. Maximum dosage is 400mg weekly. It has mood elevating properties and may worsen symptoms of agitation.

Fluphenazine decanoate
As the plasma clearance half is 2.5 to 16 weeks, individualised dose adjustment is required and the slow decline in plasma levels means that doses can be given every 2-4 weeks.

Initially, 12.5 mg is given intramuscularly. The dose is adjusted according to individual response. The usual dose range is 12.5-100 mg every 2 to 6 weeks. Interestingly, 25mg fluphenazine every 6 weeks and every 2 weeks produces similar side-effects, symptom relief and relapse rates, but with reduced drug exposure with the longer dosage interval. Fluphenazine should be avoided in patients suffering from depression and is associated with a high incidence of EPS.

Fluspirilene
This is a diphenylbutylpiperidine depot. Injection site abscesses can be prevented by sterilising the area and injecting 1-2 mls of air ahead of the fluspirilene in order to create an air pocket, which will reduce local inflammatory reactions. Initial dose is 2mg weekly, increasing as required by 2mg per week. Maintenance dose is 2-8 mg weekly. Maximum dose is 20mg weekly.

Pipothiazine palmitate
This is a piperidine phenothiazine. It is administered in doses of 12.5-50 mg weekly every 4 weeks. It is purported to have a lower incidence of EPS.

Table 3

Depot	Duration of action	Peak	Rate limiting half life	Time to steady state
Flupenthixol	3-4 weeks	7-10 days	8 days	10-12 weeks
Fluphenazine	1-3 weeks	6-48 hours	6-10 days (single doses)	6-12 weeks
			14-100 days (multiple doses)	6-12 weeks
Fluspirilene	1.5 weeks	2 days	7-10 days	5-6 weeks
Haloperidol	4 weeks	3-9 days	18-21 days	10-12 weeks
Pipothiazine	4 weeks	9-10 days	14-21 days	8-12 weeks
Zuclopenthixol	2-4 weeks	4-9 days	17-21 days	10-12 weeks

Atypical Antipsychotics

Atypical antipsychotics have a different receptor binding profile to conventional antipsychotics which may partly explain their propensity to cause less EPS and their broad range of action, namely in the management of the positive, negative and cognitive symptoms of schizophrenia. The greater tolerability of atypicals facilitates better medication compliance, which leads to better therapeutic outcomes. Atypicals are more expensive than conventional antipsychotics, but the direct and indirect savings facilitated by better medication compliance in terms of expenditure on health care and lost productivity and fewer side effects outweigh the high costs of these medications.

Atypical antipsychotics are now the recommended first line treatment for all patients with schizophrenia. Should the clinical circumstances be favorable they should be prescribed for patients experiencing first episodes or relapses of illness and for patients requiring maintenance therapy.

Amisulpiride

Amisulpiride is a substituted benzamide which binds selectively and has a high affinity to D2/D3 receptor subtypes, though it is devoid of actions at the D1, D4 and D5 receptor subtypes. It has no affinity for serotonin, alpha-adrenergic, histamine H1 and cholinergic receptors. At low doses it preferentially blocks pre-synaptic D2/D3 receptors producing dopamine release responsible for its disinhibitory effects. This atypical pharmacological profile may explain it's antipsychotic effect at higher doses through post-synaptic receptor blockade and it's efficacy against negative symptoms at lower doses, through pre-synaptic receptor blockade. In addition, the reduced tendency to produce extrapyramidal side effects may be due to its preferential limbic rather than striatal anti-dopaminergic activity. In terms of it's pharmacokinetics, the drug is weakly metabolised and is largely eliminated unchanged in the urine.

For acute psychotic episodes, oral doses between 400 and 800mg/day are recommended. Doses above 800mg/day have not been associated with greater efficacy and have induced higher rates of extrapyramidal symptoms. For patients with predominantly negative symptoms, oral doses between 50mg/day and 300mg/day are recommended.

Clozapine

Clozapine is a dibenzodiazepine and it's pharmacological profile differs from other atypical antipsychotics in many respects. It has low affinity for D1, D2, D3 and D5 receptors, but shows high affinity for D4 receptors and has potent antiserotoninergic, noradrenolytic, anticholinergic, antihistaminic and arousal reaction inhibiting effects. The reasons for clozapine's increased efficacy and low EPS are not clear. Some ascribe it to its combination of low D2 and high D4 affinity, others to its high 5HT2:D2 ratio.

The absorption of orally administered clozapine is 90-95%. It is subject to a moderate first pass metabolism, resulting in an absolute bioavailability of 50-60%. Clozapine is almost completely metabolised before excretion. Approximately 50% of the administered dose is excreted as metabolites in the urine and 30% is excreted in the faeces.

It is the drug of choice in treatment resistant schizophrenia, where it has been shown to be effective in relieving both positive and negative symptoms in approximately 30% of patients. In addition, improvement in some of the aspects of cognitive dysfunction has been described. In most patients antipsychotic efficacy can be expected with 200 to 450 mg/day in divided doses. The total dose can be divided unevenly, with the larger portion at bedtime. A few patients may require larger doses to obtain maximum therapeutic benefit. Judicious increments are permitted up to a maximum dose of 900mg/day. The risk of agranulocytosis (1% of treated patients) is dose-independent and is highest in the first year of treatment, hence the need for weekly full blood counts for the first 18 weeks of treatment. After week 18, twice weekly full blood counts are monitored until week 52, if blood results have been satisfactory. After week 52, monthly full blood counts are monitored, if a stable hematological profile is seen. If an abnormality in white cell or neutrophil count is detected then, depending on the severity of the abnormality, the clozapine is either stopped immediately or clozapine is continued and bloods repeated until the abnormality resolves. In addition, compared to other neuroleptics, clozapine is associated with a dose dependent risk of seizures. Other adverse effects include excessive salivation and sweating

Olanzapine

Olanzapine is a thienobenzodiazepine and has a chemical structure similar to clozapine. It shows high affinity for 5HT2 a receptors and a D2 affinity that is less than that of haloperidol but greater than that of clozapine. It also binds strongly to $\alpha 1$ and $\alpha 2$-adrenergic, histaminergic and muscarinic receptors. Olanzapine dispersible tablet is bioequivalent to olanzapine coated tablets, with a similar rate and extent of absorption. It is well absorbed after oral administration, reaching peak plasma concentrations within 5 to 8 hours. It is metabolised in the liver by conjugative and oxidative pathways.

The recommended starting dose is 10mg per day, administered as a single daily dose without regard for meals. Daily dosage may be subsequently adjusted on the basis of individual clinical response within the range of 5-20mg daily. It is as effective as haloperidol in the treatment of positive symptoms and appears to be superior to haloperidol in the treatment of the negative symptoms. It is associated with few EPS and to cause minimal elevation of prolactin. The most common side effects are sedation and weight gain; others include dizziness, postural hypotension and possibly abnormal glucose metabolism.

Quetiapine

Quetiapine, like clozapine, binds strongly to 5HT2 receptors and has relatively lower D1 and D2 affinity. It also exhibits antihistaminergic and $\alpha 1$ binding with moderate $\alpha 2$ adrenergic activity. Its clinical efficacy is comparable to that of haloperidol and chlorpromazine in the treatment of both positive and negative symptoms. It has a clearance half life of 7 hr, is bound to plasma proteins (83%), is extensively metabolised by the liver so that only 5% of the parent compound is excreted in the urine or faeces.

Doses need to be increased gradually over several days initially, and a starter pack is available. The Cochrane review concluded that although quetiapine is more effective than placebo, no difference could be detected against traditional antipsychotics and drop-outs due to adverse effects were lower with quetiapine, but still high. Quetiapine has also been associated with lens changes, therefore slit-lamp or direct opthalmoscopic examination is recommended at baseline and every six months during treatment with it. Starting dose is 50mg daily on day 1, 100mg daily on day 2, 200mg on day 3, 300mg on day 4. All doses are given in 2 divided doses. The usual dose is 300-400mg daily to a maximum dose of 750mg daily.

Its propensity to produce EPS appears remarkably low across the dose range. It is not associated with sustained elevation in prolactin levels and consequent endocrine changes. Common side effects include dizziness, hypotension, somnolence and weight gain. Despite being structurally related to clozapine there is no need for haemtalogical or ECG monitoring.

Risperidone
This is a benzisoxazole derivative. Risperidone is a selective monoaminergic-antagonist with a high affinity for both serotonergic 5HT2 and dopaminergic D2 receptors. Like clozapine, it is a more potent 5HT2 antagonist than a D2 antagonist. Risperidone also binds to α1 adrenergic receptors and with lower affinity to H1 histaminergic and α2 adrenergic receptors. Risperidone has no affinity for cholinergic receptors. It is completely absorbed and rapidly distributed after oral administration, reaching peak plasma concentrations within 1 to 2 hours. It is metabolised into an active metabolite in the liver. Higher plasma concentrations and slower elimination of risperidone occurs in the elderly and in renal insufficiency.

Two meta-analyses of clinical trials comparing risperidone to haloperidol suggested that risperidone may be more efficacious in the treatment of positive and negative symptoms and has a reduced risk of EPS. Its affinity for D2 receptors is greater than that of clozapine however, which may account for the dose related EPS that become more pronounced above a dosage of 6mg/day. Most patients will benefit from daily doses between 4 and 6 mg/day, although in some, an optimal response may be obtained at lower doses. The maximum dose is 16 mg daily. Dose related increases in prolactin levels are also seen and have been associated with sexual dysfunction.

There is growing evidence for the role of poor cognitive function (especially poor working memory) in poor outcome in schizophrenia and risperidone has been shown to produce an improvement in cognitive function.

Ziprasidone

Ziprasidone is a benzisothiazolylpiperazine. It has a high 5HT2a: D2 receptor binding ratio. It binds strongly to 5HT2a and 5HT2c receptors and has considerable affinity for dopamine D4 receptors. Its affinity for $\alpha2$ adrenergic receptors as well as for histaminergic and muscarinic receptors is low suggesting that its potential to produce sedation is also low. It also differs from other available neuroleptics in its blocking of noradrenaline reuptake and its 5HT1a-agonist properties.

Peak plasma concentrations are reached in 6-8 hours. Plasma half-life is 5-10 hours and steady state is reached by the third day and twice a day dosing is optimal. The usual daily dose is 80 to 160mg. Ziprasidone has many metabolites, most of which are inactive. Ziprasidone is principally metabolised by the liver.

Initial results from clinical trials indicate that ziprasidone has similar efficacy to that of haloperidol in the treatment of positive symptoms and may have additional antidepressant properties. In addition, it would appear to be effective in the negative symptoms and cognitive dysfunction observed in schizophrenia. Ziprasidone appears to be well tolerated, with low rates of EPS, no symptoms relating to hyper-prolactinaemia, and only infrequent reports of hypotension and dizziness. Ziprasidone has not been clearly associated with clinically significant hematological toxicity or ECG changes though it does prolong the QT interval.

Conclusion
Whilst conventional antipsychotics are useful in the treatment of positive symptoms their adverse effect profile is less than desirable. Atypical agents offer a broader spectrum of action though are not free of side effects. The development of intramuscular preparations of atypical agents will be welcome as it will, hopefully, obviate the need to use conventional agents in those patients in whom compliance is an issue.

References

American Psychiatric Association. 1996.
Practice Guidelines for management of patients with schizophrenia.
APA Press, Washington, DC, USA.

Davis JM, Matalon L, Wantanabe MD, *et al.*
1994. Depot antipsychotic drugs: place in therapy.
Drugs, 47: 741-773.

Glassman AH, Bigger JT Jr.
2001 Antipsychotic Drugs: Prolonged QTc Interval,
Torsade de Pointes and Sudden Death.
Am J Psych 158: 1774-1782.

Kane *et al.*
Clozapine for the treatment resistant schizophrenic.
Arch Gen Psych 1988, 45: 789-796.

Kapur S, Remington G. 2000
Atypical antipsychotics.
Br Med J, 321(7273): 1360-1361.

O'Reilly JG, Agis SA, Ferrier IN *et al.* 2000
QTc interval abnormalities and psychotropic drug therapy in
psychiatric patients.
Lancet 355(9209): 1048-1052.

Taylor DM, Mc Askill R. 2000
Atypical antipsychotics and weight gain-a systematic review.
Acta Psych Scand, 101: 416-432.

Adverse effects of anti-psychotic medication

Antipsychotic medication can cause a broad spectrum of adverse effects, some of which are medically significant. Even the minor adverse effects are important because the unpleasantness for the patient may reduce the compliance with taking medication. Many of these are the result of pharmacological effects on neurotransmitter systems in regions other than the target site for the intended thera-peutic benefits of the medication. The pathophysiology of some adverse effects have not been clearly elucidated (e.g. neuroleptic malignant syndrome). Differences in receptor binding characteristics of antipsychotic drugs result in different side-effect profiles.

Adverse effects will be discussed in the following categories:
General
Neurological – extrapyramidal and neuroleptic malignant syndrome.
Neurological – non-specific
Cardiovascular
Endocrine
Hepatic
Dermatological
Haematological
Ophthalmic
Sexual

Sedation

This is a common side effect reported by 88% of patients treated with antipsychotic medication. Sedation is mediated through H1, D2 and alpha-1-adrenergic receptor antagonism and these sedative effects of medication can be utilised in situations whereby rapid tranquillisation is required. It is important to distinguish between anti-psychotic adverse effects including sedation, depression and disease related negative symptoms of schizophrenia.

Management:
- Slow titration of dose of drug.
- Dose reduction.
- Avoidance of polypharmacy.
- Change to antipsychotic with less sedative profile

Anticholinergic effects

Dry mouth, constipation, impaired accommodation causing blurred vision, urinary hesitancy or retention and ejaculatory inhibition are ascribed to anticholinergic activity of medication. Some of the above effects are also mediated by antiadrenergic mechanisms. Paralysis of accommodation can precipitate closed-angle glaucoma. Dryness of the mouth can cause stomatitis and long term dental caries and gum disease.

Management:
- Symptomatic relief of individual symptoms.
- If severe or recurrent, change to a different class of antipsychotic medication.

Weight gain

Excessive body weight gain occurs in up to 50% of patients receiving long term antipsychotic medication. The extent of weight gain varies by drug, which may reflect the receptor binding characteristics of individual drugs. In a meta-analysis of 81 studies of weight change after 10 weeks of treatment with a range of anti-psychotic drugs, weight gain was associated with all antipsychotic drugs except for ziprasidone and molindone. Clozapine was associated with the greatest weight gain of 4.45kg at 10 weeks although there is no single mechanism responsible for this effect. Weight gain associated with medication tends to be greatest in the early treatment phase and only plateaus 4 years later. Experimental data suggest that drugs stimulate appetite by interacting in the lateral hypothalamus with dopaminergic, serotoninergic and hista-minergic receptors. Each drug has different affinities for specific receptors and thus different weight gain liabilities. Sedative effects of medication can lead to less activity and less caloric utilisation. It appears that weight gains of 5% of body weight or greater during the adult lifespan are associated with increased risks of cardio-vascular disease, cancer and diabetes.

Management:

- Dietary advice and moderate levels of exercise are recommended.
- If weight gain is problematic, consider drugs with fewer propensities to weight gain.
- Amantadine, a dopaminergic agonist, which counteracts hyper-prolactinaemia, has been used in clinical trials to manage weight gain, though caution is required as it may exacerbate psychotic symptoms.

Extrapyramidal side effects

These can be broadly divided into acute and chronic categories. Acute extrapyramidal side effects are signs and symptoms that occur in the first days and weeks of antipsychotic medication administration, are dose dependent and are reversible upon medication dose reduction or discontinuation. These include parkinsonism, dystonia, akathisia and neuroleptic malignant syndrome. Approximately 60% of patients who receive acute treatment with conventional antipsychotic medication develop clinically significant extrapyramidal side effects.

Parkinsonism

Characterised by the symptoms of idiopathic Parkinson's disease, rigidity, tremor, akinesia and bradykinesia, it results from blockade of D2 receptors in the nigrostriatal pathway and the effects can be found in 20% of patients treated with typical antipsychotic medication. Symptoms of medication-induced parkinsonism need to be carefully distinguished from negative symptoms of schizophrenia or depressive symptoms.

Management:

- Reduce medication to minimal effective dose.
- Anticholinergic antiparkinsonian medication, such as benzhexol, is effective. These lead to additional risk of developing anti-cholinergic side effects and cognitive impairment, especially in the elderly. The need for anticholinergic medications should be re-evaluated after the acute phase of treatment is over and when changing the dose of anti- psychotic medication as anticholinergic medication may no longer be necessary.

Dystonia

Acute dystonia is characterised by the spastic contraction of discrete muscle groups. Dystonic reactions occur in 10% of patients initiating therapy and 90% of reactions occur within the first 3 days with the neck, eyes and torso most commonly affected. Risk factors are young age, male gender, use of high-potency medications, high doses and intramuscular administration.

Management:
- Responds well to anticholinergic medication given parenterally. Prophylaxis of further episodes with oral anticholinergics.

Akathisia

Characterised by somatic restlessness that is manifest subjectively and objectively in 20%-25% of patients treated with conventional antipsychotics Characteristically patients complain of an inner sensation of restlessness and an irresistible urge to move various parts of their bodies. Objectively this presents with increased motor activity. This is extremely distressing to the patient and is a cause of noncompliance with medication.

Management:
- Reduce the dose of the medication.
- Switch to a different antipsychotic.
- Anticholinergic antiparkinsonian medication has limited efficacy unless the patient has concurrent parkinsonian symptoms.
- Centrally acting ß blockers e.g. propranolol, may prove useful.
- The evidence to support the efficacy of benzodiazepines in acute akathisia is largely anecdotal.

Neuroleptic Malignant Syndrome

This is not a true extrapyramidal side effect but an idiosyncratic drug reaction that can occur with all antipsychotic drugs. It is included here because extrapyramidal motor disturbance is a cardinal feature of this rare and potentially lethal syndrome.

Characterised by the triad of rigidity, hyperthermia and autonomic instability, including hypertension and tachycardia, it is often associated with an elevated serum creatine kinase level. The patient is often confused and demonstrates altered consciousness. The prevalence is uncertain and may occur in as many as 1%-2% of patients treated with antipsychotic medication. The syndrome has been reported to occur with lithium.

The pathophysiology has been explained by a central hypodopamin-ergic state. A recent paper suggests that the taqI A polymorphism of the dopamine D2 receptor gene is associated with a predisposition to the syndrome.

Risk factors include young age, male gender, pre-existing neuro-logical disability, physical illness, dehydration, rapid escalation of dose, use of high-potency medications and use of intramuscular preparations.

Management:

- Early recognition and intervention are necessary to prevent mortality. Discontinue the medication and transfer to a medical unit to provide supportive treatment for the hyper-thermia and cardiovascular symptoms. Bromocriptine, a dopamine agonist, accelerates reversal of the condition. Dantrolene promotes muscular relaxation. Antipsychotic rechallenge following NMS is associated with an acceptable risk in most patients. Treatment is resumed with a lower-potency antipsychotic medication than the precipitating agent, with gradually increased doses.

Chronic extrapyramidal side effects are signs and symptoms that occur after months and years of antipsychotic medication administration, are not dose dependent and may persist after medication is discontinued.

Tardive Dyskinesia

This is a hyperkinetic abnormal involuntary movement disorder caused by sustained exposure to antipsychotic medication that can affect neuromuscular function in any region. Eighty per cent of cases involve the muscles of the lower third of the face giving rise to involuntary activity in the tongue. Tremor is not considered to be part of the syndrome. These stereotypies can be combined with grinding/chewing lateral and/or anteroposterior jaw movements and puckering/pursing movements of the lips. The combination of these signs is referred to as the buccolinguomasticatory (BLM) triad. Stereotypies can be quite complex causing the patient to march on the spot or cross and uncross their legs. Dystonic movements can be seen in the facial muscles and in head, neck and trunk muscles. Internal muscles of the oropharynx, larynx, diaphragm and intercostals may be affected with consequent effects on respiration and swallowing. Approximately 4% of schizophrenia patients will develop tardive dyskinesia for each year of continuing medication. The majority develops mild symptoms with approximately 10% developing severe symptoms. Risk factors include older age, female gender and postmenopausal status, concurrent medical disease especially diabetes mellitus, diagnosis of an affective disorder and use of high doses of antipsychotic medications. It is important to consider that spontaneous dyskinesias occur in drug naïve patients, though the prevalence is much higher in patients treated with antipsychotics. The pathophysiology has not been fully elucidated.

The post-synaptic dopamine receptor supersensitivity hypothesis may be an oversimplification. It may involve increased dopaminergic and noradrenergic activity and disrupted GABAergic and cholinergic activity in the pathways between the substantia nigra and basal ganglia to the thalamic and subthalamic nuclei. Tardive dyskinesia may arise after exposure to any antipsychotic medication except clozapine. We do not have, to date, sufficient data on all the atypical antipsychotic medications in clinical use to draw firm conclusions about their risk of causing tardive dyskinesia.

Management:
- Primary prevention must be the focus for practising psychiatrists.
- This entails prescribing antipsychotic medication for psychotic disorders only, prescribing the minimal effective dose and avoiding polypharmacy.
- When tardive dyskinesia occurs, discontinuation of medication may alleviate symptoms but this course of action is often not clinically possible.
- Stopping medication may exacerbate the symptoms.
- Atypical antipsychotic medication, especially clozapine, is beneficial.
- Avoiding concurrent use of anticholinergic medication and anti-depressant medication improves outcome.
- Vitamin E (alpha tocopherol) has been reported to reduce symptoms though results are not unequivocal.
- The other management options include benzodiazepines, propranolol, clonidine, bromocriptine and the dopamine depleting drugs such as tetrabenazine.

Neurological Adverse Effects (II)

Seizures

Almost all antipsychotic drugs alter the EEG. There is a general slow-ing of waveforms, a decrease in alpha waves and an increase in gamma and delta waves. Paroxysmal discharges similar to epilepti-form activity may be seen. These electrophysiological changes lower the seizure threshold. There is approximately a 1% risk of anti-psychotic drugs precipitating seizures. Past or family history of epilepsy, or pre-existing cerebral pathology predisposes the individual to seizures. Polypharmacy, rapid increments and high-dose regimes increase the risk. Low potency conventional antipsychotic medication and clozapine pose the greatest risk. Clozapine is associated with a dose-related risk of seizures. The overall seizure rate is 2.8%. With low-dose treatment (<300 mg/day) the risk is 1%, with medium doses (300-599 mg/day) the risk is 2.7% and with high doses (>599 mg/day) the risk is 4.4%.

Management:
- If antipsychotic medication is indicated, switch to an alternative drug and addition of an anticonvulsant may be warranted.

- Consider prophylactic sodium valproate to patients thera-peutically requiring high doses of clozapine.

- Avoid using carbamazapine with clozapine, as this combination increases the risk of haematological side effects and carbamazepine reduces plasma clozapine levels.

Cardiovascular

Electrocardiographic changes and tachyarrhythmias:
Changes in the ECG include prolongation of the QT interval, which indicates delayed ventricular repolarisation. ST depression, T wave flattening and emergence of U waves may be found. A comprehensive review of the epidemiological literature suggests that the corrected QT interval (QTc) is an imprecise marker of the risk of tachyarrhythmias especially if prolonged >500msec. The association between QTc prolongation and mortality has been identified in patients with cardiac disease but is unclear in patients without cardiac disease. As stated before, prolongation of the QT interval (QTc) over 500msec may be associated with an increased risk of tachyarrhythmias, particularly of torsade de pointes. This is a potentially fatal arrhythmia. Although pimozide, sertindole, droperidol and haloperidol have been documented to cause torsades de pointes and sudden death, the most marked risk is with thioridazine. There is no association with olanzapine, quetiapine, or risperidone. Ziprasidone is associated with a mild to moderate prolongation of the QT interval, but as yet there is no evidence to suggest that this leads to torsade de pointes or sudden death.

Management:
- Baseline ECG assessment should be considered in patients with pre-existing cardiac disease.
- If cardiac symptoms such as palpitations, vertigo, syncope or seizure occur, then the possibility of an arrythmia should be considered and a cardiac evaluation, including ECG, should be performed.
- A prolongation of the QTc interval to greater than 450msec or to greater than 25% over that in previous ECGs may warrant telemetry, a cardiology consultation and dose reduction or discontinuation.
- Avoid high dose neuroleptic medication especially in those with pre-existing heart disease.
- Monitor levels of potassium and magnesium as it is important to avoid electrolyte imbalance.
- Avoid concomitant administration of medications known to prolong the QT interval.

Postural hypotension
Caused by the antiadrenergic effects of medication. If severe it can lead to syncopal episodes. This adverse effect may lead to tachycardia.

Management:
- Avoid intravenous administration of low potency phenothiazines.
- Patients should be cautioned about getting up quickly from lying or sitting positions.

Endocrine

Hyperprolactinaemia
All conventional antipsychotics increase prolactin secretion by blocking the inhibitory actions of dopamine on lactotrophic cells in the pituitary gland. This action also reduces the release of luteinizing hormone and follicle-stimulating hormone. Risperidone, an atypical antipsychotic, can cause a dose-related hyperprolactinaemia. In women, symptoms include menstrual irregularities (oligomenorrhea) or amenorrhoea in 20%, galactorrhoea in 1%-5% and breast enlargement. Impotence and gynaecomastia may occur in men.

The gynaecomastia is more related to disturbances in oestrogen:androgen ratios.

Management:
- Reduction in medication dose may decrease the severity or alleviate the symptoms.
- Change to an atypical antipsychotic medication.
- If symptoms are severe and medication cannot be changed, low doses of bromocriptine or amantadine may be used with caution as these medications may exacerbate symptoms of schizophrenia.

Osteoporosis
This condition, characterised by decreased bone mineral density, has been reported to occur in patients with schizophrenia. The accelerated decrease in bone mineral density can be partially attributed to drug-induced hyperprolactinemia. A chronic hyperprolactinemia may be associated with hypogonadism in both males and females which in turn increases the risk of osteoporosis.

Abnormal Glucose Metabolism

Antipsychotic-induced hyperglycaemia was first reported in 1964. There have been many case reports in the literature reporting drug-induced hyperglycaemia and type II diabetes, the prevalence of which has been reported as 36% in a group treated with clozapine. A review of published case reports concluded that clozapine and olanzapine are the most likely atypical antipsychotics to be linked with hyperglycaemia. However, diabetes is more prevalent in those with a diagnosis of schizophrenia than in the general population and is more common in untreated patients, thus creating a debate about the aetiology of abnormal glucose metabolism in schizophrenia.

Management:
- Monitoring blood glucose is important prior to commencing treatment and during follow-up.
- Dietary advice can control weight gain that increases the risk of developing diabetes.
- Changing the medication and addition of oral hypoglycaemic agents may become necessary.

Hepatic

Minor, transient increases in hepatic enzymes are not uncommon with antipsychotic medication. Cholestatic jaundice has been noted to occur in 0.1% -0.5% of patients taking chlorpromazine, which usually presents in the first month of treatment.

Management:
- If jaundice occurs, discontinue medication and prescribe another antipsychotic.
- It is important to rule out other causes of jaundice.

Dermatological

Cutaneous reactions occur infrequently with antipsychotic medications although an erythematous hypersensitivity-type rash can occur in 5% of patients on chlorpromazine. Photosensitivity is most common with the low potency conventional antipsychotics, as are pigmentary changes in exposed areas of skin.

Management:
- Discontinue medication and give antihistamines to treat allergic reactions.
- Advise patients to avoid direct sunlight and to use sunblock creams whilst on conventional antipsychotics.

Haematological

Inhibition of leucopoiesis can occur with use of antipsychotic medications. Such effects include a benign leucopenia in 10% of patients and the more serious agranulocytosis, which is potentially fatal. This is rare with phenothiazines and occurs in 1% of patients on clozapine. Conventional antipsychotic drugs appear to produce direct bone marrow suppression while the agranulocytosis associated with clozapine is mediated through immunological mechanisms. Increasing age, female gender and a pre-treatment neutrophil count less than 3500/mm³ increase the risk of agranulocytosis with clozapine.

Management:
- A high index of suspicion is important if patients on clozapine, especially if commenced recently, present with symptoms of infection and a white cell count less than 2000/mm³ (neutrophil count <1000mm³).
- Agranulocytosis is usually reversible if clozapine is discontinued immediately.
- Monitoring is improved by mandatory inclusion in a monitoring service (CPMS).
- When agranulocytosis develops, intensive management of sepsis is imperative.
- Granulocyte colony stimulating factor is used to accelerate granulopoietic function.
- Clozapine should not be recommenced.

Ophthalmic

Pigmentary retinopathies and corneal opacities can occur with chronic administration of the low-potency antipsychotics, thioridazine and chlorpromazine. High dose thioridazine is associated with retinitis pigmentosa and consequent impairment of vision.

Management:
- Do not prescribe high doses of thioridazine (see cardio-vascular effects).
- Patients treated with chlorpromazine and thioridazine should have ophthalmic examinations every two years whilst ideally avoiding long term use of these medications.

Sexual

Erectile dysfunction is reported in 23%-54% of men on antipsychotic medication. Loss of libido and anorgasmia are reported in men and women. Retrograde ejaculation has been reported with risperidone and thioridazine, the effects being due to antiadrenergic and antiserotoninergic effects. Priapism has been reported, although rarely.

Management:
- Dose reduction or switching to another class of antipsychotic usually results in symptom improvement.
- It is important to question patients regarding these symptoms as information may not be readily volunteered.

In summary, antipsychotic medications can cause a broad range of adverse effects, which can interfere with treatment in a number of ways. The manifestations of the side effects can limit the psychiatrists' use of a particular drug or mask treatment response as well as affecting the patient's compliance with the prescribed medication. It is, therefore, important to be aware of the range of adverse effects associated with each drug you use in clinical practice.

References

Wallace M.
Real progress – the patient's perspective.
Int Clin Psychopharm 2001; 16 (Suppl 1): S21-4.

Fenton M, Coutinho ES, Campbell C.
Zuclopenthixol acetate in the treatment of acute schizophrenia and similar serious mental illnesses (Cochrane Review).
Cochrane Database Syst Rev 2001; 3: CD000525.

Barnes TR, McPhillips MA.
How to distinguish between the neuroleptic-induced deficit syndrome, depression and disease-related negative symptoms in schizophrenia.
Int Clin Psychopharm 1995; 10 (Suppl 3): 115-21.

Lucas VS.
Association of psychotropic drugs, prevalence of denture-related stomatitis and oral candidiasis.
Comm Dent and Oral Epidem 1993; 21: 313-316.

Baptista T.
Body weight gain induced by antipsychotic drugs; mechanisms and management.
Acta Psych Scand 1999; 100: 3-16.

Allison DB, Mentore JL, Heo M, *et al.*
Antipsychotic-induced weight gain: A comprehensive research synthesis.
Am J Psych 1999; 156: 1686-1696.

Henderson DC, Cagliero E, Gray C, *et al.*
Clozapine, diabetes mellitus, weight gain, and lipid abnormalities: A five-year naturalistic study.
Am J Psych 2000; 157: 975-981.

References

Casey D, Zorn SH.
The pharmacology of weight gain with antipsychotics.
J Clin Psych 2001; 62 (suppl 7): 4-10.

Stanton JM.
Weight gain associated with neuroleptic medication: a review.
Schizo Bull 1995; 21 (3): 463-472.

Suadicani P, Hein HO, Gyntelberg F.
Weight changes and risk of ischaemic heart disease for middle-aged
and elderly men: an 8-year follow-up in the Copenhagen
Male Study. J Cardiovasc Risk 1997; 4: 25-32.

Barnes-Josiah D, Potter JD, Sellers TA, *et al.*
Early body size and subsequent weight gain as predictors of breast
cancer incidence.
Cancer Causes Control 1995; 6; 112-118.

Sakurai Y, Nakamura K, Sakurai M, *et al.*
Relationship between weight change in young adulthood and the risk
of NIDDM: The Sotetsu Study.
Diab Care 1997; 20: 978-982.

Correa N, Opler LA, Kay SR, Birmaher B.
Amantadine in the treatment of neuroendocrine side effects of
neuroleptics.
J Clin Psychopharm 1987; 7; 91-95.

Chakos MH, Mayerhoff DI, Loebel AD *at al.*
Incidence and correlates of acute extrapyramidal symptoms in first
episode of schizophrenia.
Psychopharm Bull 1992; 28: 81-86.

References

Rapniak NM, Jenner P, Marsden CD.
Acute dystonia induced by neuroleptic drugs.
Psychopharm (Berl) 1986; 88: 403-419.

Braude WM, Barnes TRE, Gore SM.
Clinical characteristics of akathisia: a systematic investigation of
acute psychiatric inpatient admissions.
Br J Psych 1983; 143: 139-150.

Fleischhacker WW, Roth SD, Kane JM.
The pharmacologic treatment of neuroleptic-induced akathisia.
J Clin Psychopharm 1990; 10: 12-21.

Cunningham DG, Owens DG.
A guide to the extrapyramidal side-effects of antipsychotic drugs.
Cambridge 1999.

Pope HG, Keck PE, McElroy SL.
Frequency and presentation of neuroleptic malignant syndrome in a
large psychiatric hospital.
Am J Psych 1986; 143: 1227-1233.

Suzuki A, Kondo T, Otani K, Mihara K, *et al.*
Association of the Taql A polymorphism of the dopamine D2 receptor
gene with predisposition to neuroleptic malignant syndrome.
Am J Psych 2001; 158: 1714-1716.

Taylor D, McConnell D, McConnell H, Abel K, Kerwin R.
*The Bethlem & Maudsley NHS Trust Prescribing Guidelines
(5th Edition), 1999.*

Tarsy D, Baldessarini RJ: Tardive Dyskinesia.
Am Rev Med 1984; 35: 605-623.

Kane JM, Smith JM. Tardive dyskinesia:
prevalence and risk factors, 1959-1979.
Archives of Gen Psych1982; 39: 473-481.

References

Bednar MM, Harrigan EP, Anziano RJ, Camm AJ, *et al.*
The QT interval.
Prog Cardiovasc Dis 2001; 43(5 Suppl 1): 1-45

Reilly JG, Ayis SA, Ferrier IN, *et al.*
QTc-interval abnormalities and psychotropic drug therapy in
psychiatric patients.
The Lancet 2000; 355: 1048-1052.

Glassman AH, Bigger JT JR.
Antipsychotic Drugs: Prolonged QTc interval, torsade de pointes, and
sudden death.
Am J Psych 2001; 158: 1774-1782.

Halbreich U, Palter S.
Accelerated osteoporosis in psychiatric patients:
possible pathophysiological processes.
Schizo Bull 1996; 22: 447-54.

Mir S, Taylor D.
Atypical antipsychotics and hyperglycaemia.
Int Clin Psychopharm 2001; 16: 63-73.

Mukherjee S, Decina P, Bocola V, Saraceni F, *et al.*
Diabetes mellitus in schizophrenic patients.
Compr Psych 1996; 37: 68-73.

Alvir JM, Lieberman JA, Sufferman AL, *et al.*
Clozapine induced agranulocytosis: incidence and risk factors in the
United States.
N Eng J Med 1993; 329: 162-167.

Pollack MH, Reiter S, Hammerness P.
Genitourinary and sexual adverse effects of psychotropic medication.
Int J Psych Med 1992; 22: 305-327.

Psychopharmacological Management of Schizophrenia

Introduction

"Primum Non Nocere" or "first do no harm" should be the guiding principle when prescribing any treatment to patients. There are many reasons why what we do as physicians may be less than ideal for our patients, for instance, using incorrect doses and multiple medications unnecessarily. Therefore, with respect to schizophrenia, polypharmacy should be avoided and clinicians should strive to minimise their patients cumulative lifetime exposure to neuroleptics by careful practice of evidence based prescribing guidelines, hence reducing the risks of iatrogenic neurotoxicity due to inappropriate usage of neuroleptics.

Investigation and Differential Diagnosis of Schizophrenia

Before prescribing, when one is faced with the management of a patient presenting with symptoms suggestive of an acute exacerbation of schizophrenia, one must first confirm that these symptoms meet DSM-IV or ICD-10 criteria for the diagnosis of schizophrenia by conducting a full psychiatric and general medical assessment. Investigations should include various blood tests, an electroencephalogram and a CT brain scan, to rule out non-psychiatric causes. In addition, it is important to assess for co-morbidity (e.g. a patient with schizophrenia having another psychiatric or physical disorder) and rule out whether the patient has an illness other than schizophrenia e.g. affective psychosis, substance misuse, personality disorder and delirium due to a medical condition or drug induced delirium. (Table 1).

Table 1

Psychiatric Illness	Non-Psychiatric Illness
Schizophreniform Disorder	Temporal lobe epilepsy
Acute and transient psychotic disorders	CNS neoplasm/trauma/stroke Delirium
Delusional Disorders	Neurosyphilis
Schizotypal Disorder	HIV
Drug-induced psychosis	Herpes encephalitis
Mania	SLE
Psychotic depression	Huntington's Disease
Personality Disorder	Wilson's Disease
Factitious Disorder	Metachromatic Leukodystrophy

Practical psychopharmacology of schizophrenia

The next section will discuss the management of first episode, acute on chronic relapse, maintenance treatment and treatment resistant schizophrenia. Once the diagnosis of schizophrenia, be it a first episode or an acute relapse, is confirmed then one must consider why this patient is presenting with psychotic symptoms at this time.

In the case of an acute relapse one should check for psychosocial stressors that may be exacerbating the patient's symptoms and for noncompliance with medications due perhaps to poor insight or to side effects of antipsychotic therapy. A good collateral history is helpful in confirming the history and assessing compliance and ongoing social stressors and supports. One must next decide whether to admit the patient voluntarily or involuntarily for observation and treatment. This is especially important if there is risk of harm to self or others or self neglect. Whatever the decision about admitting a patient, there is clear evidence that the duration of untreated psychosis determines time and degree of recovery and influences risk of relapse, hence the need to commence the patient on antipsychotic therapy once the diagnosis of schizophrenia has been established.

In selecting an antipsychotic (Table 2) the choice is of either an atypical or a typical antipsychotic. A low therapeutic dose of a single antipsychotic agent is started initially. In patients who are on other medications e.g. enzyme inducing drugs like carbamazepine, it is important to be aware of the potential for interactions with antipsychotic therapy. In elderly patients, who are more susceptible to toxicity, drug interactions and extrapyramidal side effects due to impaired renal, hepatic and cardiovascular function, doses of antipsychotics may need to be reduced. If the patient is a first episode patient then an atypical antipsychotic is recommended as a first line option. It is associated with fewer extrapyramidal symptoms (EPS) which may promote compliance and improve long term outcome and has a broad spectrum of action being efficacious for positive, negative and cognitive symptoms.

If the patient is presenting with an acute exacerbation of chronic schizophrenia one must carefully review the clinical notes and select either a typical or atypical antipsychotic that has been used effectively and been tolerated in the past by that particular patient.

As it can take up to 4 to 6 weeks for psychotic symptoms to respond to antipsychotics, the temptation to rapidly escalate the antipsychotic dose should be resisted. The symptoms that tend to respond quickly are those associated with agitation and aggression though psychotic symptoms per se can take up to 6 weeks, if not longer, to disappear. If after 6 weeks there is little change, then consider a small increase in the dose, noting that high doses are of little benefit and there is an increased risk of neurotoxicity which may lead to irreversible side effects like tardive dyskinesia.

On occasion, patients with symptoms of agitation and behavioural disturbance require adjunctive medication. Short term (8-12 weeks, including the tapering off period) use of benzodiazepines, such as lorazepam (up to 4 mg per day), can be considered.

Table 2
**Atypical and Typical
Antipsychotics-Recommended Dose Ranges**

	Dosing	Starting Dose (mg/day)	Maintenance Dose Range (mg/day)	Max Dose (mg/day)
Amisulpiride	BD	400-800mg	50-200mg (neg) 400-800 (pos)	800mg
Chlorpromazine	QDS	25mg	75-300mg	1000mg
Clozapine	BD	12.5mg	300-600mg	900mg
Flupenthixol	BD	6mg	6-18mg	18mg
Haloperidol	BD	1.5mg	3-10mg	20mg
Olanzapine	Daily	10mg	5-20mg	20mg
Pimozide	Daily	2-4mg	2-12mg	20mg
Quetiapine	BD	50mg	300-400mg	750mg
Risperidone	Daily	2mg	4-8mg	16mg
Sulpiride	BD	400-800mg	200-2400mg(pos) 200-800mg(neg) 400-600mg(mixed)	2400mg
Thioridazine	QDS	30-100mg	600mg	800mg
Trifluperazine	BD	10-15mg	10-25mg	45mg
Ziprasidone	BD	80mg	40-160mg	160mg
Zuclopenthixol	TDS	20-30mg	20-60mg	150mg

In summary, ensuring the correct diagnosis, determining whether a patient has co-morbidity, conducting physical investigations and obtaining a collateral history are as vital as ensuring that a patient gets treatment promptly. Atypical antipsychotics are to be favoured over conventional agents due to their greater efficacy (i.e. positive, negative and cognitive symptoms) and reduced propensity to cause EPS. High doses should be avoided as they offer little additional effectiveness and can cause adverse effects.

It can take up to 6 weeks for clinically significant improvement to occur, therefore the usage of lorazepam for short periods may be considered. Changing dosages or medications prior to this time frame will offer little additional benefit. These guidelines are appropriate for the vast majority of patients. However, there are a small minority of patients who are severely disturbed and require emergency pharmacological treatment, termed rapid tranquilisation.

Rapid Tranquilisation

Rapid tranquilisation (RT) is necessary for the management of acutely disturbed or violent patients. There have been few well conducted clinical trials in the area though this will change with the introduction of atypical intramuscular (IM) preparations.

Reasons for disturbed or violent behaviour:

These are many and varied but can roughly be divided into the following:

1. Schizophrenia.
2. Substance misuse.
3. Physical conditions e.g. hypoxia, metabolic disorders, infections.
4. Side-effects of medication.
5. Willful or chosen behavior.

Treatment of disturbed or violent behaviour:

1. Nonpharmacological.
   i) Prevention
      a. Patients known to become disturbed for signs of such behaviour.
      b. Direct admission to a psychiatric ICU or its equivalent.
   ii) Treat the underlying cause.
   iii) 'Talking down', distraction, seclusion, use of sanctions.
   iv) Control & restraint by trained personnel.

2. Pharmacological

If the use of antipsychotic medication is required, it is prudent to choose the drug least likely to cause serious side-effects.

A. Intramuscular haloperidol can be used and the dosing regime advised by the product data sheet is as follows:

For rapid emergency treatment – 5-10 mg stat, or infrequently up to 30 mg IM. Depending on the response of the patient doses can be given every 30-60 minutes although 6-12 hourly intervals may be sufficient.

B. Zuclopenthixol acetate is associated with significant sedation, therefore caution is advised when using this medication in neuroleptic naïve patients. It may take up to 4 hours to work so adjunctive benzodiazepines are sometimes used acutely. Peak effects are seen 24-40 hours after administration and effects last up to 72 hours. Single doses are from 50-150mg and a single additional dose may be administered 1-2 days following the first but more commonly 2-3 days up to a maximum of 400mg in 2 weeks. Maintenance oral medication should be started 2-3 days after the last injection.

C. Benzodiazepines can also be used for RT due to their sedative and anxiolytic effects. In addition, they have a wide thera-peutic index. Lorazepam (up to 4 mg stat can be given but the total daily dose is approximately 8 mg) is the drug of choice as its absorption from the IM site is predictable. Diazepam is not recommended as its absorption is erratic and slow.

A combination of antipsychotic and benzodiazepine may be indicated as it may result in lower doses of the former being used thereby reducing the risk of various adverse effects. This group of patients though small in number are important as they constitute a psychiatric emergency.

Maintenance Treatment of Schizophrenia

Approximately 20% of patients with schizophrenia have a single episode. However, it is impossible to predict exactly who these patients will be. Therefore, as schizophrenia is associated with high relapse rates, it is recommended that all patients have continuation treatment. Once the patient has been stabilised on an antipsychotic, clinical recommendations until recently had been that patients remain on continuous daily antipsychotic therapy for a minimum of 2 to 5 years after diagnosis (Table 2). Recent expert recommendations, however, are suggesting that the patients remain on lifelong maintenance therapy given the chronic nature of an illness like schizophrenia. Patients and their families must be seen regularly in an outpatient setting so as to provide support, identify signs of relapse early, to encourage compliance and monitor for medication side effects.

In patients with multiple relapses due to noncompliance with oral medications, relapse may be prevented by commencing them on depot antipsychotics. The currently available depots are typical antipsychotics but it is anticipated that there will be atypical depots available in the future. Typical depots include haloperidol decanoate, flupenthixol decanoate (activating effects), fluphenazine decanoate (avoid in depression), pipothiazine palmitate (purported lower incidence of EPS), zuclopenthixol decanoate (calming and sedative effect) and fluspirilene (problems of injection site abscesses). Before commencing a patient on a depot antipsychotic, a low dose test dose should be administered 6-10 days beforehand to assess the patient's tolerability of that depot.

Patients with schizophrenia are very sensitive to psychosocial perturbations which often require comprehensive, continuous and individualised psychotherapy. Improved compliance and global functioning have been reported following cognitive therapy. Reduction in symptoms has been reported following cognitive therapy in which treatment resistant hallucinations were treated as negative automatic thoughts or the inherent illogicality of treatment resistant delusions was challenged. Patient's beliefs about illness and medication are explored and an attempt is made to modify these beliefs.

Schizophrenic patients are more likely to relapse if they are discharged to families exhibiting 'high expressed emotion' (hostility, critical comments and emotional over-involvement), especially if they were exposed to these families for more than 35 hours per week. Education of patients and their relatives about schizophrenia and its treatment represents good clinical practice and while studies have demonstrated that patients themselves benefit little from such education, it seems likely that these efforts would help the relatives of patients. Both patients and relatives are likely to benefit from the support, information and advocacy provided by voluntary agencies and all patients and their relatives should be provided with information about such agencies. In summary, the management of patients with schizophrenia requires a comprehensive assessment of the patient and the use of preferably atypical antipsychotic therapy as part of a comprehensive psychosocial package. The overall aim is to minimise side effects, promote medication compliance and target not only positive but also the disabling negative, affective and cognitive symptoms of schizophrenia in order to improve the outcome for these patients.

Compliance

In newly diagnosed patients and patients with chronic schizophrenia, compliance with psychotropic medication is a major problem. The combination of schizophrenia with alcohol and substance misuse, poor insight, positive symptoms especially grandiose or persecutory delusions and the stigmatising side effects of antipsychotics can be factors which make compliance difficult.

Compliance is enhanced by a good relationship between patient and clinician, clear information about treatment and side effects, once daily dosing, use of depots, offering incentives for compliance, better social and psychological support and minimising side effects of antipsychotics. The use of atypical antipsychotics in schizophrenia, due to their better side effect profile, should encourage compliance. Compliance therapy is based on motivational interviewing techniques. It has been shown to improve compliance with medication in patients with both acute and chronic schizophrenia. Provided one is sure about a patient's compliance and other apparent reasons for non-response, failure to respond to adequate dose and an adequate duration of treatment has been termed treatment resistant schizophrenia. Though, as we shall see, not all patients who fail to improve are 'true' non-responders.

Treatment Resistant Schizophrenia

Approximately 70% of patients will respond, in terms of their positive symptoms, to conventional antipsychotic drug usage. Yet, if a patient has not had a satisfactory clinical response to an adequate trial (therapeutic dosage for 4-6 weeks) of one neuroleptic, switching should be considered to another antipsychotic from a different chemical class for a further 6-week period.

When switching from one antipsychotic to another, dose tapering and cross titration is recommended. This involves the gradual reduction of the dose of the drug being discontinued while gradually increasing the dose of the drug being started. This reduces the risk of symptom exacerbation due to abrupt discontinuation of the original drug but does carry a risk of side effects due to having the patient on two different drugs at the same time. If a patient persistently fails to respond then one must consider whether the criteria for treatment resistance are fulfilled.

The definition of this concept is by no means universally agreed:

1. The Kane criteria are conservative and in essence state that a patient is treatment resistant if there has been no response to 3 trials of at least 2-3 different classes of antipsychotics at 500mg chlorpromazine per day for at least 6 weeks.

2. Alternative criteria for treatment resistant schizophrenia are met if a patient remains unresponsive, or if the patient is intolerant of other antipsychotics due to disabling tardive dyskinesia, after an adequate trial of two different antipsychotics at doses of at least 1g chlorpromazine equivalents per day for six weeks.

If a patient meets these criteria then using clozapine should be considered. Before this it is imperative to determine whether the patient is 'truly' treatment resistant or has 'apparent' treatment resistance.

Reasons for apparent treatment failure
1. Non-compliance
2. Adverse effects
3. Co-morbid substance misuse.
4. Co-morbid Axis I disorder(s).
5. Axis II disorder.
6. General medical illness.
7. Psychosocial stressors.

Provided a patient is truly non-responsive then information about the risks and benefits of commencing the patient on clozapine should be clearly discussed with the patient and his family, in order that the patient can give fully informed consent to commencing on clozapine. This atypical neuroleptic is the only treatment that has been shown to work in treatment refractory schizophrenia. It is effective against positive, negative and cognitive symptoms of schizophrenia and has antiaggressive properties and is not associated with tardive dyskinesia.

A full physical work up should be performed prior to commencing the patient on clozapine due to the potentially serious hematological, cardiovascular, autonomic and endocrinological side effects associated with it. Daily compliance with clozapine is essential so it is important to select patients for clozapine who can be expected to take it on a daily basis.

Clozapine therapy can be started on an outpatient basis though, on occasion, a patient may have to be hospitalised in order to initiate treatment. The latter option is favored by clinicians due to potentially serious side effects such as headache, drowsiness, hypersalivation, tachycardia, hypertension, myocarditis and the dose dependent risk of seizures. All patients on clozapine must be registered with the

Clozaril Patient Monitoring Service and are given a unique identification number. The starting dose is 12.5mg twice daily and the dose is increased gradually over a few weeks until a therapeutic dose of at least 300mg/day is reached. If the patient's symptoms are not responding to 600mg of clozapine per day then clozapine levels are taken and if the levels are below 350ng/l then the dose is increased to a maximum dose of 900mg per day. Because the dose independent risk of agranulocytosis on clozapine is highest in the first year of treatment, weekly blood counts are checked for the first 18 weeks of treatment, fortnightly blood counts between weeks 18-52 and monthly blood counts thereafter.

If the clozapine monitoring service detects abnormalities in the white cell count then, depending on the severity of the abnormality, the clinician is notified and either clozapine is discontinued immediately or the frequency of testing is increased to twice weekly until the white cell count abnormalities resolve. If stopping clozapine, due to it's ineffectiveness, then the dose should be reduced gradually over three months due to the risk of a rebound psychosis due to the abrupt discontinuation of clozapine.

An adequate trial of clozapine is for 1 year as even though the psychosis may remit within 6 months, cognitive symptoms may take up to 12 months to respond. If the patient has not responded to an adequate trial of clozapine and misdiagnosis, substance misuse, noncompliance and psychosocial stressors that could be interfering with progress have been ruled out, then clozapine augmentation strategies should be used.

Clozapine Augmentation Strategies

1. Combining clozapine with mood stabilisers like lithium, valproate or lamotrigine can augment Clozapine but should not be used in conjunction with carbamazepine due to increased risk of agranulocytosis.

2. Clozapine can also be combined with therapeutic doses of both typical (sulpiride, haloperidol) or atypical (risperidone, olanzapine, quetiapine or amisulpiride) antipsychotics, with careful vigilance for extrapyramidal and anticholinergic side effects.

Clozapine is the drug of choice for those with treatment refractory schizophrenia. Though efficacious in 30-50% of those who take it, it is not without significant risks. Maximum doses of clozapine can be used (with adequate blood monitoring) and augmentation with other psychotropics can be considered depending on the symptom clusters present.

Antipsychotic medication is an important part of the overall treatment package for those with schizophrenia. Conventional antipsychotics are efficacious in about 70% of those with the illness though are by and large poorly tolerated due to their propensity to cause EPS. Atypicals, though not free of adverse effects, are an appealing alternative which are effective in not only positive symptoms but in the other symptom groupings as well. Maintenance treatment is required for all patients be they first episode or not and the length of this phase is anywhere from 2-5 years though the reality is that these patients most probably require life long psychotropic medication. For those with true treatment refractory schizophrenia, clozapine is the drug of choice though it may take up to 1 year before certain features improve.

References

Baldessarini RJ, Viguera AC. 1995
Neuroleptic withdrawal in schizophrenic patients.
Arch Gen Psych, 52, 189-199.

Boyer P, Lecrubier Y, Puech AJ. 1995
Treatment of negative symptoms of schizophrenia with amisulpiride.
Br J of Psych, 166, 68-72.

Carpenter WT, Hanlon TE, Heinrichs DW *et al.* 1990
Continuous versus targeted medication in schizophrenic outpatients.
Am J Psych, 147, 1138-1148.

Chakravarti SK, Muthu PK, Naik P *et al.* 1990
Zuclopenthixol acetate: single dose treatment for acutely disturbed patients.
Current Medical Opinion Research, 12, 58-65.

Chong SA, Remington G. 2000.
Clozapine Augmentation: Safety and Efficacy.
Schizo Bull, 26, 421-440.

Conley R.R., Tamminga C.A., Bartko J.J. *et al.* 1998
Olanzapine compared with chlorpromazine in treatment-resistant schizophrenia.
Am J of Psych, 155, 914-920.

Davis JM, Metalon L, Wantanabe MD *et al.* 1994
Depot antipsychotic drugs. Place in therapy.
Drugs, 47, 741-773.

Dubin WR. 1985
Rapid tranquilization, the efficacy of oral concentrate.
J Clin Psych, 46, 475-478.

Jolley AG, Hirsch SR, McRink A *et al.* 1989
Trial of brief intermittent neuroleptic prophylaxis for selected schizophrenic outpatients.
Br Med J, 298, 985-990.

References

Kane JM, Honingfeld G, Singer J. 1988
Clozapine for the treatment resistant schizophrenic: a double-blind comparison.
Arch Gen Psych, 45, 789-796.

Leucht S, Pitschel-Walz G, Abraham D *et al.* 1999
The efficacy and extrapyramidal side effects of the new anti-psychotics olanzapine, quetiapine, risperidone and sertindole compared to conventional antipsychotics and placebo.
A meta-analysis of randomised controlled trials.
Schizo Res, 35, 51-68.

Lieberman JA, Salz BL, Johns CA. 1991
The effects of clozapine on tardive dyskinesia.
Br J Psych, 158, 503-510.

Loebel AD, Lieberman JA, Alvir JM *et al.* 1992
Duration of psychosis and outcome in first episode schizophrenia.
Am J Psych, 149, 1183-1188.

McGlashan TH, Johannessen JA. 1996
Early detection and intervention with schizophrenia; rationale.
Schizo Bull, 22, 201-222.

Meltzer H, Mc Gurk SR. 1999
The effects of clozapine, risperidone and olanzapine on cognitive function in schizophrenia.
Schizo Bull, 25, 233-255.

Reilly JG, Ayis SA, Ferrier IN *et al.* 2000
QTc interval abnormalities and psychotropic drug therapy in psychiatric patients.
Lancet, 355, 1048-1052.

Scheitman BB, Lindgren JC., Early J. 1997
High-dose olanzapine for treatment-refractory schizophrenia.
Am J Psych, 154, 1626.

Thompson C. 1994
The Royal College of Psychiatrists Consensus Statement on the use of high dose antipsychotic medication.
Br J Psych, 164, 448-458.